THE BREAST CANCER CARE BOOK

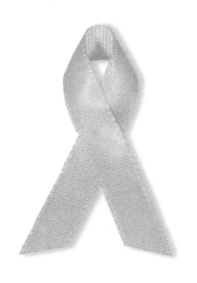

THE BREAST CANCER CARE BOOK

*A Survival Guide for
Patients and Loved Ones*

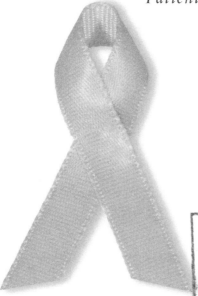

SALLY M. KNOX, M.D.

WITH JANET KOBOBEL GRANT

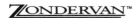

ZONDERVAN™

GRAND RAPIDS, MICHIGAN 49530 USA

ZONDERVAN™

The Breast Cancer Care Book
Copyright © 2004 by Sally M. Knox

Requests for information should be addressed to:
Zondervan, *Grand Rapids, Michigan 49530*

Library of Congress Cataloging-in-Publication Data

Knox, Sally M., 1954-
    The breast cancer care book: a survival guide for patients and loved ones / Sally M. Knox with Janet Kobobel Grant.
        p. cm.
    Includes bibliographical references and index.
    ISBN 0-310-24870-1
    1. Breast—Cancer—Popular works.   I. Grant, Janet Kobobel.   II. Title.
RC280.B8K585 2004
616.99'449—dc22

                                                                                2004001547

Interior design by Michelle Espinoza

Printed in the United States of America

---

04 05 06 07 08 09 10 /❖ DC/ 10 9 8 7 6 5 4 3

To my family—Ryan, Susan, Kathleen, Kelly, and Dianna
And to my Lord and Savior, Jesus Christ

Contents

Acknowledgments   9

PART 1: THE TRIP YOU DIDN'T SIGN UP FOR

1. The Journey Begins   13

2. Testing, One, Two, Three   27

3. Travelmates: Your Medical and Personal Support Teams   37

4. Consulting the Great Physician   55

PART 2: THE MEDICAL JOURNEY

5. What Are Your Surgical Options?   75

6. Choosing the Right Surgery for You   89

7. The Next Step: Post-Surgery Chemotherapy and Hormone Blocker Therapy   111

8. Moving Onward: Radiation Therapy   129

9. Alternative Healing Methods   141

PART 3: TRAVELING WITH FINESSE

10. Emotions: Making Them Work for You   153

11. Your Spouse, Your Biggest Supporter   175

12. Helping Children Face the Challenge   185

13. Restoring Fitness and Well-Being   193

14. After Cancer   209

Appendix A: Risk Factors   213

Appendix B: Resources   223

Notes   233

About the Authors   237

Scripture Index   239

Subject Index   241

ACKNOWLEDGMENTS

I t's hard to say enough thank-yous to the many colleagues, patients, and advisers who have made this book come to life.

Thank you to my colleagues who reviewed and contributed to this book, whose expertise is greatly appreciated: Nathan E. Williams, M.D., breast and gynecological oncologist, Asheville, N.C.; Jan Pettigrew, Ph.D., R.N., oncology and grief counselor, Little Rock, Ark.; David M. Euhus, M.D., associate professor of surgery, Division of Surgical Oncology, University of Texas Southwestern Medical Center at Dallas; Joseph A. Kuhn, M.D., surgical oncologist, Baylor University Medical Center; Joyce A. O'Shaughnessy, M.D., codirector, Breast Cancer Research, and director, Breast Cancer Prevention, Baylor-Charles A. Sammons Cancer Center, Dallas; John E. Pippen, Jr., M.D., medical oncologist, Baylor-Charles A. Sammons Cancer Center; William M. Carpenter, M.D., reconstructive surgeon, Baylor University Medical Center; Michael D. Grant, M.D., breast surgeon, Baylor University Medical Center; Michela Caruso, M.D., radiation oncology; Robert P. Scruggs, M.D., director of Radiation Oncology, Baylor-Charles A. Sammons Cancer Center; Neil Senzer, M.D., director of Radiation Oncology Research, Baylor-Charles A. Sammons Cancer Center; Marvin J. Stone, M.D., chief of Oncology at Baylor University Medical Center, director of Baylor-Charles A. Sammons Cancer Center; Kathleen Caton, manual lymph drainage specialist; Dr. Ruth Bolton, family practice, Wayzata, Minn.

Thank you to Sue Coffman, Kelley Mathews, and Sandra Glahn for their writing skills as they collected interviews and helped the survivors' stories come to life.

Kathy Latour, thanks for your encouragement, support, writing expertise, and insight, all of which helped to make this book happen.

Thank you to Andre Kole, Ed Komoszewski, Bob Tiede, and David Shibley for their contributions regarding the faith issues faced by survivors.

Thank you to Cindy Brinker Simmons for her contributions.

Gene Rudd and Barbara Snapp tirelessly nursed this along until it actually came to life. I couldn't have done it without you.

Thank you to my editor, Cindy Hays Lambert, who seemed to be there with encouragement at just the right moments.

Many survivors and families have bravely and willingly shared their experiences so others could be encouraged: Margaret E. Ashmore, Sheila M. Balagna, Brenda Bankston, JoAnn Boots, Cindy and Jim Cervine, Sandy Cranford, Bill and Jane Cutrer, Mary F. Goolsby, Josefa Iglesias, Sharon K. Mankin, Cheryllynn D. Merritt, Jyme Parish, Lola Rodgers, Jody and Dave Stevens, Patricia L. Strahm, Tonya Reynolds, Kelly and Troy Wagers, Karen White, Evelyn Williams, Deborah and Faron Young, and Nancy Rubin.

Others reviewed chapters and gave valuable insight: Dolores M. Carruth, M.D., Pamela George, Kay Hammer, and Jeannine Sandstrom.

My office staff has been invaluable to me and helped in more ways than I can count. My deepest thanks to Jan Pinkston, Deborah Young, Ruth Price, and Kris Reading for sticking with me through so many challenges. Grace Cobb helped to edit and proofread chapters. You all made it happen. Thank you.

PART I

THE TRIP YOU DIDN'T SIGN UP FOR

CHAPTER I

THE JOURNEY BEGINS

Twenty-five-year-old Tonya had experienced her share of transitions. In a little over a year she had married and was now seven months pregnant. As a nurse in an obstetrician's office, she previously had experienced the joy of a new life coming into the world with countless women. Now at last it was her turn. As she felt the baby move and kick, her mind raced ahead to the drastic changes her life would undergo in just two more months when her baby boy made his appearance. Then one day Tonya brushed across her breast and stopped a moment. Did she notice something new, a lump? *Not a lump, really,* Tonya assured herself. *It's more like a clogged milk duct.* At her next appointment with her obstetrician, she told him about it.

Next thing she knew, she was on her way to see a radiologist for an ultrasound. After imaging the area, the radiologist studied the results for what seemed to Tonya like hours.

Finally he said, "You know, I just don't believe this is malignant."

Well, that's good, Tonya thought. *I never dreamed it really might be.*

Tonya's obstetrician wanted her to see a surgeon, who recommended a mammogram followed by a biopsy.

Tonya was from a small town about eighty miles from the large city where her surgery was to be done. Since the biopsy was early in the morning, her parents took a second car so Tonya and her mom could shop for baby items when the procedure was over. Her husband and her dad would head back home. Tonya and her mom would have plenty of time after the procedure to make an event of the trip, so Tonya made a mental list of the stores she didn't want to miss.

During the biopsy, Tonya joked and talked with her surgeon. Then somebody came into the surgical suite and all conversation ended.

Tonya was puzzled when she was placed in a private alcove in the recovery room. Most patients were in a larger area with just curtains separating the beds. *They probably want to check the baby,* she surmised. Her family joined her along with her surgeon. She noticed tears in her surgeon's eyes. And then the unimaginable happened. The surgeon used the words "BREAST CANCER."

As a physician who has had to say those words to many women, I know that the first time any woman hears them, the world stops for a moment. Nobody is prepared to hear the report, even if a family member or close friend has had cancer, even if you suspected before the biopsy, even if . . . There is a world of difference between thinking *I might have cancer* and having that fear confirmed.

FIRST RESPONSES

I've found that, most of the time, patients hear little else of whatever the physician says at that time. You are numb, shocked, flooded with questions for which you want immediate answers. These are normal responses. Often women say their first thought is, *I'm going to die.* Fortunately, that isn't true. Most will recover. But the fear of death and the intrusion of a dreaded enemy eclipse everything else at that moment.

Tonya, now recovered and healthy, says, "I remember little about that time. I recall the room, and my husband, John, holding my hand. My mother held my forehead. I remember thinking, *Oh, my God, how is this possible?* My surgeon told me, 'You're going home today, and I would like to see you back tomorrow. Bring all of your questions, and we'll talk about what we need to do.' I thought that was good and bad—bad because I wanted to know right then, but good because it gave me a chance to gain some perspective."

Have you, too, felt the frightening impact of the words, "You have breast cancer"? Did you feel your life had taken a jarring turn in a dreadful direction?

Cancer is a rude travel companion, bringing with it several suitcases stuffed to overflowing with stress enhancers and expecting you to carry the luggage! It demands to have its own way and has no concern for the itinerary you had created for yourself. It doesn't care that your family has needs, that you're trying to hold down a job or advance your career, that its presence strains your relationships with those closest to you. It's indifferent to the physical, emotional, and spiritual havoc it wreaks. It sets its own schedule and pays no attention to your pleas to stop for a break.

As breast cancer's unwilling travel companion, do you feel you've lost control of all that's important to you? Do you struggle between focusing on the myriad of questions to which you want answers and concentrating on the flood of emotions you're experiencing? If so, your response is normal, I assure you.

Many women have journeyed this way before you—you are not alone. In reality you are in the company of hundreds of thousands of resilient women.

As a surgeon who specializes in breast cancer, I have had the privilege of caring for many of these women. Over my nearly twenty years in this role, I have developed tremendous respect for the women who have faced this terrifying disrupter of their lives. They have shown themselves to be women of strength, fortitude, courage, and humor. Not that they didn't feel afraid, weary, and overwhelmed many times, but my respect came as I saw them move forward through the journey, regardless of what life asked them to face.

The book you hold in your hand is designed with you in mind. Together we will explore your questions, your emotions, and—be sure to catch this next step—your *options*. Yes, you *do* have options. I plan to lay out a map for you to follow on your journey so you can look ahead to the upcoming "destinations" and find spiritual turnouts that can provide you with respite. Along the way I'll explain new terms as well as potential twists and turns. This is a book about how to care for yourself, how to trust God's care, and how to lean on the care of loved ones as you journey through breast cancer. It is a book about receiving the care you need during this time.

FACING THE EMOTIONS

Have you noticed that the rush of questions and emotions seems overwhelming? Most women in your circumstances have said the same thing. So let's start there, as we clear some of the fog that may be clouding your vision. Then we will follow with a discussion of your options.

The following responses to the pronouncement of breast cancer are typical.

Sandy, 58, found that she could say, "It is a cancer" or "It is a diagnosis of cancer." What she avoided saying was, "I have cancer."

She didn't want to feel like it was hers or a part of her. She wonders if it will be easier to say, "I had cancer."

Karen, 59, suspected something was wrong when she noticed a periodic twinge of pain in her right breast. "One night, as I was getting into bed, I thought, *I need to go into the bathroom and look at my breast.* I had never paid much attention to my body. And I never looked at myself in the mirror, despite the whole bathroom being covered in mirrors. But when I felt my breast, I could feel two lumps under the nipple, and the nipple was dimpled. I had ignored some signals I should have listened to. I immediately pulled out my medical encyclopedia and realized I probably had breast cancer.

"I took it to the Lord right away. I remember saying to him, 'I know there is nothing more I can do except seek medical counsel as soon as possible.' I asked him to take away the tumors, but I also told him that if he didn't, then I knew he had a higher purpose, and that I was willing to submit to his will."

A mammogram the next day confirmed Karen's fears.

Karen felt she had ignored the signs of a problem and had to deal with guilt. "I had to just confess it and ask God to forgive me. There wasn't anything I could do about it now. I also knew that I wouldn't have been able to prevent cancer. I just might have found it sooner."

With God's help, Karen changed the guilt into conviction. Guilt lays like a heavy weight on our shoulders, and it brings no benefit with it. Conviction allows us to acknowledge a poor choice and to make a change.

THE BIG "WHY"

Discovery of breast cancer evokes questions about why, when, and how it happened. These thoughts and the feelings that accompany them are normal. In a culture steeped with cause-and-effect relationships, the patient and family often seek to find a culprit or something to blame to help make sense of all this. Was it the stress in her life? Perhaps it was the estrogen she was taking in menopause. Maybe it was her diet. She knows it was too high in fat and deficient in fruits and vegetables.

Women who eat right, exercise right, and do everything right still get breast cancer. (For more about risk factors, see Appendix A.) More is being learned every day about injuries to the cell's DNA, the "command center" of a cell that starts the problem. Damage to this command center causes the cell to do things it's not supposed to do, such as dividing uncontrollably. But while we understand more of *what* happens to an individual cell to make it go bad, no one can predict *when* or *to whom* this will happen on an individual basis. Risk factors by themselves cannot explain it. Most women diagnosed with breast cancer have no known risk factors.

Sandy's breast cancer was found when her doctor felt a lump during her annual physical. "On my doctor's desk was my normal mammogram report from the previous week," Sandy said. This made his finding all the more surprising. As her doctor explained, mammograms and physical examination of the breasts are complementary, detecting different things. Each procedure, by itself, can miss things the other technique can detect. The two together give greater accuracy. In Sandy's case, her breast tissue was dense, which meant there was little contrast between the normal breast tissue and the cancer on the mammogram. But because she followed through with an examination by her physician, the cancer was detected.

MOVING FORWARD

Women look back and scour the last year or six months for what they or someone else could have done differently to detect their cancer. While that's a normal response to a cancer diagnosis, it wastes emotional energy on something that cannot be changed. That energy is needed for the battle ahead. The best tactic is to move on and focus on winning the battle.

That is what Tonya did. Because she's from a small community, the word had spread by the time she and her family arrived home. And the word everyone received was, "It's cancer, and we hear it's bad."

Several friends had gathered at her parents' home. After offering expressions of concern, the men drifted off to find comfort in work. Eventually the women went their way as well. Tonya and her mom were left to talk. They considered the worst things that could happen: What if the baby didn't make it? What if the baby had a problem? What if the cancer was worse than they had imagined? They turned each negative over in their minds as if they were examining a complex puzzle. (The baby was born early but healthy.) Facing the fear decreased the power of the fear. You're likely to find the same is true for you, too.

Putting the cancer out on the table also allowed them to take it to God. "I think that helped us to gain perspective," Tonya said. "And it allowed us to rely on our faith as we moved forward."

God is not an intruder. Instead, he waits for us to turn to him with our hurts and questions. As we acknowledge to him our fear, anger, and doubt, we invite his response. And he never fails to respond. Even if we don't understand the answers to all our questions, God steps in. As trust grows we see, in time, that he truly has our best interests in mind and that he moves in our lives with love, kindness, and wisdom beyond our comprehension.

Tonya sat down and wrote out every question that occurred to her—and she had a lot of questions. That in itself was therapeutic.

CUSTOMIZED COPING

Identifying questions and facing your emotions are the healthiest ways to begin the journey through breast cancer. Beyond just the physical challenge, family dynamics change and emotions ride a roller coaster. You can experience a deep healing, both physically and emotionally, or give in to unhealthy patterns that become entrenched if those responses are pursued.

After learning she had breast cancer, Jody, 45, set about putting her house in order, literally. "I planned to work hard on the house and try to get the kids' photo albums and other projects completed as well as see family and friends. There's a lot I can do to prepare. I really shouldn't think of my life as being on hold as I have been since the diagnosis."

Coping patterns are as individual as the women themselves. The amount and type of information a woman wants and needs are different. Some immediately search for all possible information. They collect books, contact organizations, search the Internet, and talk to friends. Others want only the essential information immediately and prefer to seek out more details later—or never. Both are very legitimate ways of coping.

There is no one-size-fits-all mold. Ask yourself what has been helpful to you in the past. When facing challenges, do you find that a stack of books and information empower you or overwhelm you? Does being surrounded by people energize you or drain you?

You can be more resourceful than you may realize. Your spiritual background and coping skills will help you. After all, you have faced crises before. Draw strength from those spiritual and emotional sources that you've already cultivated. Recognize that each family member may take a different path to healing, and give room to those differences.

Sheila talked with her priest after she learned she had breast cancer. She asked for prayer, but she didn't tell anyone else. She didn't even tell her two grown sons right away. Then she told her youngest, who was living at home. For Sheila, waiting to tell others helped her to sort through her own feelings and emotions and to feel more in control. Eventually she did tell her church family, which provided overwhelming love and support. She found particularly thoughtful a woman who offered a spontaneous prayer for Sheila's healing.

Sharon, 40, found out about the cancer on Monday, but she didn't cry until Tuesday night. When her family was told about the diagnosis, "panic ensued." That's how she describes it. She felt she couldn't fall apart because she needed to be strong for her kids. Waiting until Wednesday to discuss it in depth with her surgeon was almost unbearably difficult for Sharon.

Lola, 62, kept her focus on the Lord. "Before I knew the results of the biopsy," she recalls, "I sat behind two friends of mine in church. One had lupus and the other rheumatoid arthritis. That put my situation in perspective for me." She had come to rely on God's Word, especially the Psalms, when she had uterine cancer two years before. She found her comfort again in Scripture. "I had learned Psalm 121 when I was a child, and as I went through the various tests, when I was on the table, I would repeat it to myself."

I lift up my eyes to the hills—where does my help come from?
My help comes from the Lord, the Maker of heaven and earth.
He will not let your foot slip—he who watches over you will not
*   slumber;*
indeed, he who watches over Israel will neither slumber nor sleep.
The Lord watches over you—the Lord is your shade at your right
*   hand;*
the sun will not harm you by day, nor the moon by night.
The Lord will keep you from all harm—he will watch over your life;
the Lord will watch over your coming and going both now and
*   forevermore.*

Jane, 45, says, "I don't think anyone ever thinks they'll get cancer despite the fact that it's all around us." After her diagnosis, she and her husband asked their church's prayer chain to pray for them. "But we asked that no one call us because we had decisions to make. That hurt some people, but I think most understood." Sometimes patients want to talk, and sometimes they don't. We should take our cue from the patient.

BEGINNING THE MEDICAL PROCESS

Once the initial shock has passed, the patient and loved ones can absorb and respond to what seems like a mountain of new information. Fortunately most women have time to seek and gather counsel before starting treatment. In most cases, you can take several weeks to educate yourself on this new challenge before entering treatment. Many patients, however, find that making a decision and moving on into treatment helps them cope and feel as if they are doing something concrete.

Let your physician guide the timing for you. In most cases a few days or a week or two won't hurt, and that time can be very helpful to you. Face your feelings and personal needs as they come. Getting numerous medical opinions is helpful, but at some point, they become burdensome and it's time to move ahead. Opinions from friends or others who have recovered from breast cancer may or may not prove helpful. What was right for a friend may not apply in your situation.

You might want to ask yourself these questions to help guide you in how to positively move forward:

- What am I afraid of?
- What questions can medical personnel help to answer for me?
- Who do I want to tell about my condition?
- How do I want to present the news?
- In what ways would a second opinion be helpful?

FACING THE FOE—TOGETHER

Realize that those who are close to you are also hurting and looking for ways to help. You need to "let them in" when that feels safe. When you are able, let them see your heart, your feelings, and your emotions. This opens up the lines of communication and helps them heal as well. Talk openly about the diagnosis, treatment, or whatever else is on your heart. Many times those close to you have been trying to act cheerful for your benefit, when they really need your permission to admit their own pain. You give them that permission by open communication and honestly acknowledging your own feelings.

Although it would seem useful to shield others from your tears and feelings, lack of communication can actually foster fear and uncertainty. The silence can suggest that the worst will probably happen. Just bringing up the topic and putting it out for honest discussion will go a long way toward dispelling that fear. This is often met with relief on the part of those close to you.

Humans by design function best in community. It will take an entire support team to get through this experience, and it's important to take the initiative in letting your team members know how they can help. Because everyone's needs are different, even people who have helped you in another situation may be uncertain about how to help without your specific guidance.

Open discussion helps in interacting with children as well. Although discussions should be tailored to the individual child and his or her maturity level, open conversation about the cancer is preferable to shielding them from the truth. Children quickly sense when "something is up." When they don't know exactly what is going on, they fear the worst. But when you allow them to be a part of your healing process, and they understand that you will honestly share with them about your treatment and what it means, they will feel more secure. This approach also gives them permission to ask questions about things you would never have anticipated they were wondering. Young children in particular will respond according to the parent's emotional tone. If you are positive and upbeat in explaining what will be happening, they will be as well. If you are fearful and negative, they will reflect that.

One of the important aspects of fighting this unseen enemy is to realize that you and your loved ones will experience grief. Loss is a close relative of cancer—the loss of a breast, the loss of control, the loss of precious time and energy. Understanding your treatment options can help give back a sense of control. And as you gain more confidence in your knowledge of what is happening and why, some of that control *is* recovered. Once you face and acknowledge the changes that breast cancer brings, emotional healing can begin. In the next chapters, we'll help to equip you for your journey by delving into a deeper understanding of what breast cancer is and what treatment options are available.

WHAT LOVED ONES CAN DO

Becoming a support person for a woman with breast cancer can be as challenging as having breast cancer yourself. You may feel it's more painful to watch someone you love in pain than to suffer the crisis yourself. You may care deeply about the situation but be uncertain how to help.

Perhaps the best overarching principle is that your presence is the most valued contribution you can make to your loved one during this time. One parent who lost a child expressed it this way:

"I was sitting, torn by grief. Someone came and talked to me of God's dealings, of why it happened, of hope

---

beyond the grave. He talked constantly. He said things I knew were true. I was unmoved, except to wish he'd go away. He finally did.

"Another came and sat beside me. He didn't talk. He didn't ask me leading questions. He just sat beside me for an hour and more, listened when I said something, answered briefly, prayed simply, left. I was moved. I was comforted. I hated to see him go."[1]

Other specifics include:

Tell her you care

Your friend with breast cancer doesn't necessarily need you to understand what she is feeling or to do anything about the details of her struggle or her treatment. Perhaps the most important thing to communicate is simply that you care about the woman and her loved ones.

Sometimes words like "I understand" sound hollow. Even if you have had exactly the same experience, what is at issue is not so much that you know how it feels as it is that you simply care about your friend. Make sure she understands that.

Be a companion

Your physical presence is a tremendously caring gesture and a great comfort.

For Lola, a friend who had breast cancer provided lots of support. "When I had my biopsy, she brought food over," Lola recalls. "She told me she had been praying it wasn't cancer. Then she helped to lighten the mood by saying she wondered if it was contagious."

Allow room for silence

No two people are alike, so be sensitive to how much conversation, if any, is wanted. Be comfortable with silence and realize that you have no idea what a deep ministry your presence is for your friend, even with nothing said. Sitting in a waiting room with your friend can be an act of caring with few or no words required, because waiting to see a physician can be scary and lonely. Your friend gets the clear message that you are there for her.

Be emotionally present

When we "rejoice with those who rejoice, and weep with those who weep," it creates a bond that gives strength to the one suffering. Advice, even good advice, is not nearly so empowering. But a friend willing to stick close by will be deeply valued.

Strengthening Thoughts
from God's Word

"In him [Jesus] and through faith in him we may approach God with freedom and confidence" (Eph. 3:12).

"Do not throw away your confidence; it will be richly rewarded. You need to persevere so that when you have done the will of God, you will receive what he has promised" (Heb. 10:35–36).

CHAPTER 2

TESTING, ONE, TWO, THREE

Part of understanding these procedures includes having a clear picture of what cancer is. We all think we know what cancer is—something about cells multiplying out of control. But our knowledge often doesn't go beyond this vague notion.

Each cell in your body is a miracle of organized activity and function, the complexity of which scientists are just beginning to understand. Thousands of cells could fit on a pinhead, yet each cell rivals a city in its complexity. The city center (nucleus) contains books that describe in great detail how every part of the city and each citizen in the city should function.

Just as in a normal city, something breaks in the cell every day. Somebody's washing machine fails, another person spills coffee on his computer. Certain people devote their entire day to finding and fixing these problems. These people determine whether the computer is so damaged that it must be replaced or whether a simple cleanup will do. Sometimes the problems are so serious that these people recommend the entire city (or cell) be shut down.

Cancer develops when a cell becomes so damaged that it needs to shut down but fails to do so. The books in the city center (the DNA of the cell) become damaged. Two pages are torn out of one of the books, a whole book is lost, or something cleverly overwrites the information in one of the books. Instead of the book reading, "The street cleaners shall sweep the streets from 1 to 2 A.M. daily," it now reads, "The street cleaners shall sweep the streets from 1 to 1 A.M. daily." This instruction is interpreted to mean the street cleaners should sweep all the time.

The fix-it people are supposed to find and fix errors before such a disaster happens. But for whatever reason, this one gets by them, throwing the whole city into disarray. The problem can't be fixed because the fix-it people can't get to work either.

This happens in a cell that becomes malignant. The DNA is damaged, but instead of the cell shutting down, it now begins to divide and duplicate itself without the checks and balances it previously submitted to. Every time it duplicates itself, each new cell has the same errant DNA, fostering a whole community of these abnormal cells.

Why do cells become malignant? The DNA repair may be less effective than it needs to be (too few fix-it men available), increasing the possibility of a problem going undetected or unrepaired. Or multiple injuries to the DNA may overwhelm the cell's repair mechanisms. No single factor explains cancer development. What we do know is that anything that damages the DNA could potentially cause cancer.

DETECTING BREAST CANCER

How do you know if you have breast cancer? As we've all heard over and over again, one of the best "tests" is simply examining your own breasts each month. That's how Kay first developed suspicions that she had breast cancer.

"We had just moved," Kay recounted. "With two young children to settle in school, boxes to unpack, a new house to make into a home, and then the holidays, my stress level was over the top. But we made it through all those events. Then, the night before we left for a long-needed vacation, I laid down exhausted. I went through my monthly ritual of breast examination more from habit than from concern. As I pushed and prodded my right breast, my fingers were drawn to a 'thing.' After years of monthly self-examination, I knew what my lumpy breasts were supposed to feel like."

Kay went to her doctor, who told her, at the age of 30, she was too young to have breast cancer. Kay insisted on a mammogram. The result? Breast cancer.

MAMMOGRAMS

Mammography was first employed in the early 1900s but didn't come into common use until the 1960s. The techniques of mammography have improved dramatically over the past forty years. As a matter of fact, the single most significant contributor to decreased death from breast cancer over the past thirty years has been earlier detection, primarily by mammograms. The American Cancer Society and other organizations recommend a screening mammogram before age 40 and then annually after 40.

What's a mammogram? An X-ray of the breast tissue done with specialized equipment. The breast is compressed (gently) between two plates to get the clearest image of the tissue with the lowest possible radiation to the breast. Most mammography units are now accredited by the American College of Radiology, which has created standards of excellence in technique, equipment, and personnel. The accreditation is voluntary and usually is stated on the patient information sheet from the mammography suite. Have your mammogram done at an accredited location so you'll be assured that the equipment and personnel meet these standards.

A mammogram may be called a "diagnostic mammogram" or a "screening mammogram." This terminology can be confusing, as the films taken are the same—usually two views of each breast. But women who have no breast complaints may have screening mammograms at a slightly lower cost because the radiologist reads them after patients have left the site. A diagnostic mammogram starts out with the same two views of each breast, but the radiologist reads them immediately and additional images are taken before the patient leaves if something is identified that needs clarifying.

I know, mammograms aren't fun—the X-ray plate surely is stuck in the refrigerator between patients, the technician dips her hands in iced water before touching you, and the squishing of your breast isn't the most pleasant of events in your day. But mammograms do save lives; so we might just as well take a deep breath and dive on into the experience.

Nancy managed to see the light side of life while getting her diagnostic mammogram. Musing that buildings and centers always seem to be named for people who died, she decided that she was going to dedicate a bathroom stall in the mammogram center to "Nancy—Who Survived Cancer and Plans to Die in Her Bed of Natural Causes When She Is 86." She suggested to her husband that if he truly loved her, he would die six months later of a broken heart. He said he would think about it.

Comparing a current mammogram with mammograms from previous years provides a great deal of information. That's one of the reasons you should have mammograms taken at the same facility each year or obtain old mammograms and carry them with you to the new center. The radiologist can request previous films with your approval, but that delays the comparison, often for several weeks.

Even though your physician will receive a report of the mammogram results, he or she usually won't have the films. So keep records about where your mammograms have been done.

Once a lump has been discovered in the breast, the first diagnostic procedure is usually a mammogram. However, some cancers are invisible even on properly performed mammograms. That means you need to see your physician if you feel a lump or a change in your breast even if your mammogram is normal. As Kay's experience shows, mammograms and a physical exam of the breast are complementary. Teamed together, they add up to a high rate of cancer detection.

ULTRASONOGRAPHY AND OTHER OPTIONS

With ultrasonography, sound waves create an image of the breast tissue, using no radiation. A sonogram gives information complementary to the mammogram rather than replacing it, but is used alone for pregnant women or young women under thirty.

MRI, CT scans, and other types of imaging have been used in breast evaluation, but they haven't reached the mammogram's accuracy. The MRI in particular holds promise as a technique, but it won't replace mammography in the near future. Instead, it might become useful in screening women at high risk for breast cancer.

TYPES OF BREAST BIOPSY

Should your mammogram indicate the need for further testing, several types of biopsies are available. Fortunately, most breast biopsies yield benign (noncancerous) results.

FINE NEEDLE ASPIRATION

Fine needle aspiration (FNA) is a popular biopsy with some surgeons and hospitals. During this procedure the doctor places a needle in the breast tissue, and cells are removed and placed on a glass slide. If fluid is obtained from the tissue, called a "cyst aspiration," the lump is resolved, and no further procedures are necessary. If no fluid is obtained, the tissue is removed through the needle and sent to a pathologist, who looks at the cells. This procedure can indicate if tumor cells are present.

However, a negative result isn't a guarantee that the area is cancer free. The needle simply might not have been placed into the tumor area. FNA is rarely the final word about breast cancer's presence. Another procedure usually will follow that produces a more certain diagnosis.

CORE NEEDLE BIOPSY

Called a "core needle biopsy," this procedure is done either by a surgeon or a radiologist in the office. The skin is anesthetized and a larger needle is used to cut out a small core of tissue and remove it. Several cores are removed and sent to the pathologist, who issues a report within a few days. This procedure removes considerably more tissue than the fine needle aspiration, but is more accurate.

Sometimes several tests are necessary before a diagnosis can be made. Cindy, for example, first had a mammogram, followed by a sonogram. But the radiologist couldn't see well behind the thickening tissue. So Cindy scheduled a needle biopsy. The biopsy revealed Cindy had cancer.

STEREOTACTIC CORE NEEDLE BIOPSY

Another type of biopsy uses a specialized digital mammography machine to identify the lesion and computer assistance to take the needle sample. This is called a "stereotactic core needle biopsy."

OPEN SURGICAL BIOPSY

Finally, an open surgical biopsy may be done. This procedure generally is done as outpatient surgery with a local anesthetic and sedation, or sometimes with a general anesthetic. An incision is made over the lump, usually about an inch in length, and the tissue is removed and examined by the pathologist.

Each of these procedures has advantages and disadvantages. The FNA is quick and simple, but might not be adequate to rule out cancer. The core needle biopsy usually renders an accurate diagnosis, but doesn't remove the entire lump in most cases. It can also be associated with significant bruising that makes subsequent evaluation more difficult. The open biopsy removes the entire lesion, but is more extensive surgery, requiring an incision.

Discuss these options with your surgeon, who can provide you information about which will serve you best. Ask your physician:

- Why is this procedure being used rather than other options?
- What does the test involve?
- How long does it generally take?
- Where is it performed (in the physician's office, the mammography center, etc.)?
- What does it feel like to have the test done?
- What sort of painkiller is used, if any?
- What are some of the aftereffects?
- When will results be available?
- Who will be giving me the results? And how will the results be given—over the phone or in the office?

Once you've received a diagnosis of breast cancer, a medical team needs to be assembled, as does a personal support team. We'll talk about how to pull both teams together in the next chapter.

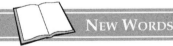

New Words

Core needle biopsy: Placement of a large needle in the breast that removes a sliver of breast tissue to be evaluated by a pathologist.

Cyst aspiration: Placement of a tiny needle in the breast that withdraws fluid and resolves the cyst.

Diagnostic mammogram: Two or more views of each breast done in women experiencing a breast problem.

Fine needle aspiration (FNA): Placement of a tiny needle in the breast and withdrawal of cells for evaluation by a pathologist.

Open surgical biopsy: A breast biopsy that entails an incision and removal of a block of tissue.

Screening mammogram: Two views of each breast done in women without breast complaints.

Stereotactic core needle biopsy: A needle biopsy that uses computer technology and mammogram images to guide the doctor in obtaining tissue from the breast. This type of biopsy requires women to lie facedown on a special table with the breast placed through an aperture in the table. The breast is gently compressed and a needle sample taken.

Ultrasonography: Sound waves used to evaluate the breast tissue. This gives complementary information to the mammogram.

WHAT LOVED ONES CAN DO

This is a pensive time for everyone involved. So far words like "probably," "maybe," "not sure" have been used. But these tests will bring more definitive answers. What can you do to support the patient?

- Be on hand when the test results are given. If the results are given over the phone, be part of the conversation, listening in on an extension line. (Let the doctor know you are there and introduce yourself.)
- Write down what the doctor says about the results.

- If words are used that neither you nor the patient understands, ask for an explanation.
- If the patient doesn't think to ask what happens next, ask the doctor.
- After the conversation, ask the patient if she wants to be alone or have you stay with her. Be sure to set aside sufficient time to be with the patient, if that's her preference.
- Don't offer Pollyanna responses such as, "I'm sure everything will turn out fine," or "Cheer up, it could have been worse." Be a listener. You don't have to offer advice or solutions.

STRENGTHENING THOUGHTS
FROM GOD'S WORD

"Be still, and know that I am God" (Ps. 46:10).

"Search me, O God, and know my heart; test me and know my anxious thoughts" (Ps. 139:23).

"I pray that you, being rooted and established in love, may have power, together with all the saints, to grasp how wide and long and high and deep is the love of Christ, and to know this love that surpasses knowledge—that you may be filled to the measure of all the fullness of God" (Eph. 3:17–19).

CHAPTER 3

TRAVELMATES: YOUR MEDICAL AND PERSONAL SUPPORT TEAMS

Breast cancer is a call to action. Once a woman learns she has cancer, she needs to assemble a team to help her forge her way through the journey ahead. It can help to think of this as an expedition that requires a team of experts and a team of travel companions. We'll explore in this chapter how to assemble your teams and what expertise each team member brings to the junket. You can approach this challenge logically and judiciously, as you would other complex issues in your life. You'll find taking a proactive role in the process is empowering.

Lola found that to be true. After telling Lola that she had cancer, her doctor said, "This will be hard for you to believe, but some people can be thankful after they've had cancer because of the benefits in their spiritual growth. You may feel that way, too."

"That gave me something to latch onto," Lola said. Realizing that the way she approached the upcoming months could make an immense difference, she concentrated on the spiritual benefit of the journey and purposefully set about putting her team together.

THE MEDICAL TEAM

Your first team consists of medical professionals who concentrate on the technical aspects of the journey. The second team, your friends and relatives, provide emotional, physical, and spiritual reinforcement. We'll first look at the professional team.

You may be surprised to find that you are about to entrust yourself not to one doctor, but to several doctors. Though the size of your medical team may vary, in many cases, it will consist of your primary care physician, surgeon, medical oncologist, radiation oncologist, plastic surgeon, and nurses. Before I describe their roles in your care, let's cover some important preparations for building your medical team.

KEEPING YOUR RECORDS STRAIGHT

Each time you see a new physician, you will be asked the details of your current problem, medical history, medications, allergies, and family history. Write out this information ahead of time, especially if you're on several medications or have previous medical problems. Each physician will request his or her own record of these details, and the information needs to be accurate.

To help you organize the mound of data that will be coming your way, I suggest you put all of your appointments on a large calendar that your family can consult. You might also include a list of doctors' phone numbers on the calendar for quick reference.

Also, set up a three-ring binder as your medical notebook. Set up tabs for:

- Questions to ask at your next appointment with each doctor.
- Test results.
- Prescription records. List drugs, dosages, and dates of prescriptions and refills.
- Resources (home-care nurses, medical supply stores, etc.).
- Phone list of medical personnel and directions to each location.
- Phone record. List to whom you talked, what was communicated, and the date. This record can be especially handy when you want to double-check with your doctor that you understood directions his nurse gave you over the phone or what tests you need to take before your next doctor's appointment. Also, it will provide you with reminders of names of receptionists and other office personnel.
- Funny things. This list will help to remind you that even in dire circumstances, humorous events can provide relief from the intensity of the situation.
- Medical history. Writing out your history will help you to recall details you might forget when you meet with new members of your team.
- Instructions. When a number of instructions or complex instructions are given, you'll feel more secure if you write down the information rather than rely on your memory. This section also provides a reference for you when you are attempting to apply a medication or treat a side effect at home.

- Doctor visits. In this section, you'll record what transpired at each doctor's appointment. It will free you from having to try to recall dates or the order in which procedures were undertaken.
- Finances. Keep invoices, reports from your health insurance, and other aspects of the financial side of your journey in this section.

Retaining this information in one spot will enable you to respond to emergencies with efficiency, to have a resource you can turn to for details you no longer remember, and to give you the assurance that you are following instructions. The more responsibility you take for listening carefully and informing yourself, the more confidence you will gain.

Preparing for a Medical Appointment

When you make an appointment with a new physician, a member of the office staff will inform you of items you need to bring, such as X-rays and reports. It will save time and frustration if you have all the information available for that first visit.

Don't be intimidated by the medical aura. If you have a question or concern about any test, medication, or treatment being offered, speak up. Physicians or nurses might not realize you don't understand something. Asking gives them the opportunity to clarify and build trust and rapport. Open communication reduces stress, and studies show that an active, problem-solving approach to conquering breast cancer hastens recovery.

If you take a few days to research doctors, that time delay will not have a negative effect on your battle against breast cancer. Your primary physician is a good source for recommendations of others to join your medical team, especially if you have had a long and trusting relationship with him or her. Your doctor will be more aware of the type of physician with whom you would relate well. Also, ask friends, family, and breast cancer survivors you may know for recommendations. See if a particular name keeps coming up.

That approach worked for Cindy, who called a friend as soon as she found out about her diagnosis. That friend mentioned a surgeon in her church who specialized in breast cancer. Then Cindy talked to a neighbor, who recommended the same surgeon, saying the surgeon had performed a cyst aspiration for her. When another friend, who oversaw a number of breast cancer recovery groups, recommended that same surgeon, Cindy made an appointment with that doctor. "There's no other doctor I would go to," Cindy recalls deciding. "She wasn't a provider with my insurance company, but my insurance paid 100 percent anyway." (I'd recommend you settle this issue up front with your insurance company, should you find a doctor who isn't part of your plan. Cindy's experience is not typical.)

LOCATION: ONE OF YOUR FIRST DECISIONS

Determining whether to use a large, comprehensive cancer center in a major city or a hospital closer to home and a local team of physicians is challenging. There is no simple answer, and no one answer is right for everybody. Each situation has advantages.

The larger cancer center will likely be involved in various research studies. Is that something that appeals to you? Anywhere you are treated for cancer, the choice to participate in research is entirely yours, but more studies typically are available at the larger centers. At large cancer centers, students or residents (physicians in training) often are involved in your care under the supervision of experienced attending physicians. Some patients like that because it gives a "cutting edge" feel to their care. Others prefer the more personal touch being closer to home.

Cancer is a serious diagnosis, so it may warrant forgoing surroundings you're comfortable with or that are more convenient for top-of-the-line care. In a comprehensive cancer center, your main assessment of physicians will involve rapport. The system in place at such institutions will get you to a highly qualified individual who can treat your cancer. The question is whether you can work with these people and the system on a long-term basis. In a smaller town, make a reasoned assessment of the physician's qualifications. Some of the most skilled surgeons I know practice in small towns.

DOING YOUR FACT-FINDING

When you call a physician's office, consider asking all or at least some of these questions:

- Is the physician board-certified in surgery or oncology or in whatever specialty he or she is practicing?
- What additional training has he or she had?
- What are his or her primary practice interests?
- How many surgeries of the type you need has he or she done?
- Ask to talk to patients who have used this physician. Are they pleased?
- How much experience does this physician have with breast cancer?
- Does he or she belong to medical organizations associated with cancer treatment?
- Does your insurance cover treatment with this doctor?

If the receptionist or other office personnel are reluctant to answer these questions, you might be wise to consider looking elsewhere for a doctor. None of these queries are unusual or inappropriate, but instead show you are being careful and thoughtful about the decision you must make. You are in control of this part of the process and should trust your instincts.

Brenda, for example, chose a surgeon based on a friend's experience with that doctor. When the friend was told she had breast cancer, the surgeon, realizing the woman was alone and had driven quite a distance for the appointment, offered to let the woman spend the night in her home. Brenda knew that kind of personal concern was what she wanted in her surgeon—in addition to skill as a surgeon, of course.

DURING THE FIRST APPOINTMENT

When you first meet a physician, you are stressed and not at your best. Your first impression of a doctor won't necessarily be representative of how your rapport will develop. The physician is learning your style and personality, and you are learning his or hers. If the initial encounter seems strained, you may want to give it another chance, especially if this person is highly qualified and you would like to stay with him or her. In a large city, you may have numerous options and prefer to move on. Don't feel guilty if you have given the relationship a reasonable chance, but the chemistry just isn't right. You need to feel good about your doctors.

The shock and emotional stress of a cancer diagnosis are debilitating for most patients. This is normal. Hearing and comprehension are impaired. So take one or two people with you for consultations with physicians. Almost without exception, spouses or friends fill women in on details they don't recall.

Because you are under so much stress, you may feel that, in seeking a second opinion, you obtain more information from the second physician. That may be the case. But you would feel that way even if the second physician said exactly what the first one said. By the time you see the second physician, you have had more time to recover and can absorb more information. Expect that and take it into consideration when making decisions. If the first and second doctors' recommendations are similar, you will feel more confident about treatment options. If the opinions differ, you become aware of potential areas of controversy, which you can then research.

You might not feel the need for a second opinion, and that's fine. But consider sitting down with your doctor a second time or recording the first consultation, knowing that you won't absorb it all. Also, if circumstances permit, pick up a book on breast cancer or research breast cancer on the Internet prior to the consultation. Reading this book will help to prepare you for how your journey in fighting breast cancer will unfold, and I've provided additional resources at the back of the book. With the knowledge you gain from your research, you will find yourself hearing much more of what the doctor says because the discussion won't be completely foreign to you.

Once you are satisfied with doctors and treatment choices, don't let the comments of others make you second-guess. Have confidence in your decision.

Now, let's take a look at the specific personnel who will make up your medical team.

PRIMARY CARE PHYSICIAN

The primary care physician is the "travel guide," if you will, of your medical group. This physician will be in charge of overseeing your map to health. Both patient and physician need to feel satisfied with the relationship. Good communication between you and your doctor fosters confidence and clarity—you have agreed on the basics of the journey. Doctors want their patients to understand their treatments and should encourage and assist them during the information-gathering stage. It might be helpful for you to realize that doctors continually assess how much information a patient and her family want and tailor the discussion to suit the patient. Do you want to know each part of the itinerary and the details of the entire trip? Or do you want the overview and to entrust the specifics to your physician? If you want more information, never hesitate to ask—but be prepared to hear the truth.

The other members of your cancer treatment team normally communicate with your primary care physician, but as you collect your reports, you can also provide specific details and copies of reports to your primary physician. He or she may be the most important member of the team, serving as a counselor and overseer of all the treatment methods. Throughout treatment, you may have a number of health issues not specifically related to your cancer that your primary physician can address with you. For example, primary physicians can be invaluable resources for hormonal issues that come up, both during and after treatment.

SURGEON

A surgeon may be the first doctor to evaluate you after a problem with your breasts comes up. The surgeon is trained to evaluate breast problems and will want to review both your breast exam and any studies that have been made, such as a mammogram or sonogram. When you make your appointment, the surgeon's office should be able to inform you of the doctor's credentials, including factors such as board certification and years in practice. Surgeons who have received specialized training for malignant diseases are called "surgical oncologists." Other general surgeons may have completed additional study specifically pertaining to breast evaluation or may limit their practices to patients with breast problems. The most important criterion is to find a surgeon who is up-to-date and does a lot of management and treatment of women with breast problems. That surgeon could be a general surgeon, a surgical oncologist, or a breast specialist.

At the outset, the surgeon should discuss to your satisfaction what problem is being evaluated and what diagnostic and treatment options are available, including risks and benefits. The specifics of the procedures should be covered, including length of surgery, recovery time, and when to expect a report after the procedure. The surgeon should encourage your questions and not feel threatened if you want a second opinion. You should feel that your surgeon respects you and treats you courteously. Offering that same respect back to him or her fosters a healthy working relationship.

Unfortunately, Sandy didn't find that to be her experience, and it alerted her to the need to change surgeons. During her first appointment, the physician recommended a needle biopsy. She reassured Sandy not to worry. Five days after the biopsy, Sandy met with her surgeon to discuss the results. Breast cancer. Sandy felt the physician had set her up with false expectations and then went about explaining the test results in a way that made it harder for Sandy to handle. This sort of beginning is hard to overcome in the doctor-patient relationship.

MEDICAL ONCOLOGIST

A medical oncologist is a physician who specializes in treating cancers with chemotherapy or hormonal therapy. These doctors have been trained in internal medicine and then have completed several additional years of training to treat cancer. Women, including those with small or early breast cancer, will want to see a medical oncologist after surgery to get his or her insight into whether additional therapy is appropriate.

Your surgeon or primary physician usually will refer you to a medical oncologist. Selecting a medical oncologist is just as important as selecting the right surgeon because this is another relationship that will continue for several years. Since communication among your surgeon, primary physician, and medical oncologist is important, you may want to stay within your doctors' recommendations. But your rapport is important. Move on if you are uncomfortable with the doctor recommended. You may be able to get another name from your referring doctor.

RADIATION ONCOLOGIST

A radiation oncologist is a physician who plans and implements radiation therapy. Women who elect to have a lumpectomy, and some who have a mastectomy, will see a radiation oncologist. The radiation oncologist will discuss the risks and benefits of radiation in your particular situation and determine the timing, dose, and specifics of treatment. Again, communication, as well as skill, is important.

Jody felt that the radiation oncologist was the "most clear about what is facing me" of all the physicians she initially saw. "We [Jody and her husband] were impressed with him in every way. He had studied my particular situation and clearly gave all the pros and cons. Dave and I left the appointment having made the decision for a lumpectomy with radiation." Jody and Dave felt their decision was a solid one because of the straightforward and understandable consultation they had with the radiation oncologist.

PLASTIC SURGEON

A plastic surgeon or reconstructive surgeon may become involved if a woman chooses to have a mastectomy with either immediate or delayed reconstruction. Breast reconstruction can be done several ways, some of which are more involved and complicated than others. The best person with whom to discuss the various procedures and to help determine which is best for you is a plastic surgeon.

NURSES

Most of the specialists you see—the surgeon, medical oncologist, and radiation oncologist—may have nurses working with them who have a high level of expertise in that doctor's specialty and can be an enormous help. These are specialists in their own right and often can clarify something a physician said that you might not have understood. Nurses are an excellent source of support, encouragement, and information. Make an effort to get to know them and utilize their knowledge.

Deb is a highly skilled nurse who works for a surgeon who treats breast cancer. She consistently takes patients "under her wing" to make sure they get personal attention for all their concerns, medical and otherwise, during treatment. Kelly relied on Deb throughout her cancer treatment. "Deb said that this whole thing is 90 percent attitude and only 10 percent physical. I remember laughing with Troy, my husband, because my whole life I've been told I had an 'attitude.' I guess this time that was a positive thing! Deb will never know how many things she said to me that carried me through the six months I was on treatment. Time and again, she accurately predicted what my next challenge would be, shared funny stories with me, and encouraged me. I used her counsel as a road marker all the way through."

COUNSELORS

Finding a counselor who can help you and your family weather the emotional storm of breast cancer can be helpful as well. Cancer puts stress on family relationships, and each family member will handle that stress differently. Having a professional to talk to can be an important way to find healthy responses. A number of resources are available to cancer patients including psychologists, pastors, social workers, and others who have had training in helping patients cope with cancer. Your physicians will be familiar with the resources available to you. Make full use of these people. Often they can make the difference between misery and thriving through and after the treatment. They can direct you to support groups and serve as skilled "listening ears" with reassurance and wise counsel. As with any other professional, rapport and honesty are important.

When you have your first conversation with a counselor, as with the other members of your team, feel free to ask questions to determine if this is a good fit for you. You might ask:

- Does he or she have experience in counseling cancer patients and their families?
- What professional training does the person have?
- How many years of experience?
- What part does this person feel faith has in the coping process? Is his or her view compatible with yours?
- Do you feel comfortable in telling this person what you're thinking and feeling?

If you don't sense a good connection with this person and don't believe he or she can help you to cope, then you haven't found a good match. Don't give up; try another counselor.

Feeling overwhelmed and reeling after reading about the medical team? Don't be alarmed by the number of choices you have to make. Think in terms of taking one step at a time. Having a lot of choices means you have a lot of control. And remember, you aren't the first woman to walk this path. To put all this into perspective, women report that one of the most stressful periods in the breast cancer experience is the time between diagnosis and the beginning of their treatment. We'll take a closer look at each treatment in greater detail in upcoming chapters; so, for now, just try to absorb the basics rather than feel you have to comprehend all the details.

PERSONAL SUPPORT TEAM

In addition to all the medical professionals, you'll want to assemble a personal support team. Think in terms of the gifts, abilities, and passions each potential team member might contribute. One person may be a dedicated "pray-er"; another quick to offer more tangible help, such as cleaning your house, doing laundry, or cooking meals. Others may be available to go with you to your treatments and to wait with you in the doctor's office. Another person may be your "professional" encourager, available to be "on call." This person would tend to know when to listen, when to offer advice, and when just to pray with you. Do you know a natural delegator, someone who can get others organized and moving? That person could creatively solve a variety of problems for you that you don't have the energy to deal with. Babysitting, running errands, answering the phone for you, doing yard work, reading to you when you don't feel well enough to read yourself, are possible ways people can support you.

List areas where others can provide support and then ask a person to be responsible for each area. That individual doesn't have to do all the labor of, say, cleaning your house, but he or she could commit to either doing it or finding others who will. When someone asks how he or she can help, you can pull out your list and let your friend decide how to be involved. Most people will be grateful for the specific direction, and you will feel more organized.

Think about using a journal as a place in which you can confide all your hopes, dreams, fears, and prayers. It can be a wonderful outlet and a source of comfort and encouragement should you later choose to share it with others facing difficult battles in their lives.

Many women form a prayer group around them or utilize a "ready-made" group they were already involved in to offer regular prayer. The patient communicates with this group through email, phoning one person, or praying with the group, depending on her inclination or physical ability at various times. Praying gives those who live in other parts of the country something concrete they can do to support you. And knowing others are praying will be a comfort to you.

Your personal and professional teams can't make the nightmare of cancer disappear, but they can smooth the path before you—and save your life. Consider each person carefully before "recruiting" them to be on your team. Trust your instincts and ask God for direction. These are the people who will form your network during your intense and highly personal journey through breast cancer. They are your companions whose care for you and your welfare will deepen in significant and profound ways as the journey unfolds. They are God's gift to you.

Speaking of God, he's on this journey with you as well. In what ways can this experience deepen your relationship with him? How do you resolve some of the spiritual questions that arise when faced with the fearful specter of cancer? We'll take a look at those questions and more in the next chapter.

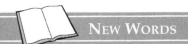

New Words

Chemotherapy: Drugs usually given through an IV targeted toward cancer cells.

Hormonal therapy: Drugs that block estrogen or progesterone, usually given orally once a day.

Radiation therapy: High doses of radiation given to the breast or chest wall to kill cancer cells.

Red Light, Green Light

Keeping these thoughts in mind will help you to select a medical team that suits you.

The relationship with a doctor is likely to work if . . .

1. You have good communication on the first appointment.
2. You feel comfortable expressing your questions and concerns.
3. The doctor has the ability to explain to you in language you understand what is happening with your body.
4. You feel comfortable with the doctor's qualifications and have confidence in his or her medical ability.
5. You relate well to the doctor's support staff.
6. The doctor isn't impatient with your questions.
7. You feel you could cry in front of the doctor and not be uncomfortable.

The relationship is unlikely to work if . . .

1. You feel the doctor is in too big a rush to adequately answer your questions.
2. The doctor seems impatient with you when you try to explain how you feel.
3. The doctor doesn't seem able to communicate medical information in a way you can understand.
4. The support staff is brusque and unhelpful, especially when you call the doctor's office.
5. You feel the doctor isn't as compassionate as you need.
6. You have concerns about the doctor's ability to perform the necessary medical procedures.
7. The doctor is offended if you want a second opinion.
8. The doctor and you do not experience mutual respect.

STRENGTHENING THOUGHTS
FROM GOD'S WORD

"It is God who arms me with strength and makes my way perfect"
    (2 Sam. 22:33).

"The Lord upholds all those who fall and lifts up all who are bowed down" (Ps. 145:14).

"For God did not give us a spirit of timidity, but a spirit of power, of love and of self-discipline" (2 Tim. 1:7).

WHAT LOVED ONES CAN DO

Jane, a breast cancer overcomer, offers this helpful advice to loved ones:

"Spiritually, everyone handles a cancer diagnosis, treatment, and follow-up differently. Almost all will at some time ask God, 'Why?' If they voice that question to you, they probably don't expect or even want an answer. The best response is, 'I don't know.'

"I have a friend who is a young believer and has thyroid cancer. One of the older saints of the church told her the reason she had cancer was because she had unconfessed sin in her life. Not very helpful!

"Most patients are looking for simple support. This isn't a time to quote Romans 8:28 to them—they have to conclude for themselves, in their own way, in their own time, that all things (including cancer) work together for good.

"That's not to say that a cancer diagnosis and treatment is a spiritual wasteland. On the contrary, it often is a time of closeness to God because you must trust him and depend on him in ways you never have before. But that has to be learned and experienced on an individual basis.

"Tell the patient you're praying for her, and then do so—in her presence and after you leave."

Kelly, who developed cancer when she was 36, found her husband provided loving support by going with her for her tests and treatments. Sometimes she wanted to talk about a procedure or how she felt, but he didn't want to hear the details. Despite his own feelings, he listened because he knew that's what she needed.

Tonya felt fortunate that a friend's mother, who had overcome breast cancer, showed Tonya her scars and told her some of the details of what Tonya could anticipate. Tonya felt that was a "life link" that helped her to accept what the future might hold.

Toppy appreciated her family as never before after her cancer diagnosis. Her husband and three daughters presented her with a poster board the night before surgery. "They had planned a calendar to begin the day after surgery with pictures of my support team of family and friends. Each day the calendar's page showed the ones who were 'on duty' to take care of me, and what special treatments and appointments with doctors were to occur. They called it 'Attack the Cancer.' My surgery went well. I was home from the hospital two days later. With such an awesome group of doctors and nurses, I have continued to get better and better as each day goes by. I thank God every day for blessing me with all these special people in my life."

CHAPTER 4

CONSULTING THE GREAT PHYSICIAN

Taking care of oneself spiritually is an integral part of a woman's journey through breast cancer. Many women have gone before you and are cheering you on, knowing that once the physical battle is under way—and sometimes even when it's over—the harder work of experiencing spiritual healing begins. The struggle often is uncomfortable because cancer never makes sense. How can a good God allow cancer? Life's realities can seriously mess up our theology.

You might manage to push tough questions aside for a time, sometimes burying them for years without resolving the issues cancer raises. In such situations, most of us struggle to escape the grip of those difficult questions. But, if we're fortunate, eventually we'll lose the wrestling match and find ourselves left only with our heartfelt issues as we stand before our Creator. All pretenses have fallen away. In this broken-down condition, we are awed to find God waiting, calmly attentive, welcoming us to bring our hurts, misunderstandings, sufferings, and questions in childlike simplicity to him. He longs to dress our wounds, to offer comfort, and to guide us to healing. God isn't threatened by our questions; he welcomes and uses them.

God is the source of the love, security, and strength that are needed. He alone understands how you feel, what your journey through cancer is like for you. Even someone who has had a similar experience can't know completely what you're going through. He alone knew you before you came into this world and knows the spiritual journey he wants to take you on. His love is personal, specific, and intimate. His love has the power to take you to your next step. Nothing else really can.

RECOGNIZE YOU ARE WEAK

How do you press close to God at such a time? Every woman is unique, and no two people will heal the same or walk exactly the same path. But one thing we have in common is our weakness. The very weakness we resist allows him to show himself strong. In 2 Corinthians 12, Paul admits to the readers of his letter that he had a "thorn" in his flesh that forced him to face his weakness. Paul proclaims, "Three times I pleaded with the Lord to take it [the thorn] away from me. But he said to me, 'My grace is sufficient for you, for my power is made perfect in weakness.' Therefore I will boast all the more gladly about my weaknesses, so that Christ's power may rest on me" (vv. 8–9).

We all tend to dislike weakness in ourselves. We hide it as best we can by appearing to be "in control." But cancer can be an opportunity to turn control over to another, to someone bigger and stronger than yourself. When you do, God moves in his way and in his timing. Are you ready to turn your cancer over to him, or are you still bargaining with him? Will you trust him only if you can make sense of all of this or if you see progress in your recovery? Or will you simply trust him? No strings attached. No bargains, no guaranteed outcomes. Simple trust requires considerably more effort and commitment than handling matters yourself, but the reward is much greater too.

Most of us wonder how to genuinely live a life of faith when the journey through breast cancer has exhausted us physically, emotionally, and spiritually. What we need to do can be stated simply: We need to trust. But how do we make that happen in our lives— every day, even the hard days?

FOCUS ON GOD

A good place to start is to focus your attention on who God is and on what he has said in his Word, the Bible. Jesus serves as a good example for us. When he faced a terrible death on the cross, he focused on the joy he knew was coming. The writer of Hebrews suggests, "Let us fix our eyes on Jesus, the author and perfecter of our faith, who for the joy set before him endured the cross, scorning its shame" (Heb. 12:2). When Paul was in prison he worshiped and focused on the joy of knowing God. After being severely beaten and thrown in jail, "about midnight Paul and Silas were praying and singing hymns to God" (Acts 16:25). Facing breast cancer or any stress of that magnitude takes you to the Lord. It may be precisely the thing that causes you to grow and mature in your relationship with your Savior.

Focusing on the Lord and his strength is not the same as smiling on the outside while crying on the inside. David, throughout the psalms, brought his feelings and questions to God. At times he was joyful, other times despairing. But he always was honest. That humble genuineness opened the door to David's heart and let the Lord do what seemed best. And the same can be true for you.

When God gave us our emotions, he intended us to experience them. Tears need to be cried to bring healing. Healthy ventilation of emotions helps us to process the events and circumstances that are taking place. Once the painful emotions are vented, it's possible to move on and to focus on the Lord and his truth. Venting and then refocusing are both components of healing. But be sure your venting isn't destructive; don't attack others or place blame.

YIELD TO GOD'S WAY

Sometimes we resist what God is teaching us or resist following him down the path he wants us to walk because it involves suffering. That's normal. When you recognize this happening, stop and yield your heart again. You don't have to like what is happening, just be willing to take the next step before you. The richness of your relationship with Jesus can become far more significant than the cancer that caused you to need him so badly.

Dr. Keith Willhite, a professor at Dallas Theological Seminary, learned several lessons about God as he suffered through his medical challenge. "I had few symptoms, so my physician's announcement that I had a brain tumor came out of nowhere," writes Dr. Willhite. "My wife, Denise, and I prayed together for a few minutes. Then I left the room to pray alone.

"I acknowledged to God that He is both good and sovereign, and my life is in His hands. But I also told Him I couldn't imagine why He would call me to heaven and leave a young widow with two small children. It was difficult, but I tried to pray, 'Your will be done.' I also prayed that God would give me a doctor who is a fighter....

"As I rested for several weeks after my two brain surgeries, I had many hours to ponder the 'why' questions. Why is God allowing this suffering in my life? Is there a specific sin? Am I sure? If not, then is there something God wants me to learn? Am I so out of focus that He needed to take me to this point so I will trust Him more? Maybe you have wondered the same questions."[1]

BE CONFIDENT IN WHO GOD IS

Dr. Willhite found that the reason for suffering might not be clear. Not knowing can be frustrating. But the experience taught him that God is trustworthy. Confidence that God is good alleviates some of the struggle and puts the weight on God's shoulders. It frees the heart and mind to simply deal with the circumstances at hand without guilt and without fear that God is frowning or unhappy with us. In many ways, when we face a medical calamity, we are like a child who needs stitches after a bad cut. If that child believes the doctor is his friend and isn't angry with the child for hurting himself, he can relax and let the physician inject the numbing medicine and stitch him up. That injection stings, and because he may be too young to understand it all, he could think that the sting is because someone is mad, when that isn't the case at all.

Confidence that God is trustworthy, compassionate, and not disappointed with us counts most when we suffer. That assurance regarding who God is may be harder to hold onto during times of stress, but calling to mind truth from the Bible helps us to focus. Go to the Scriptures that have meant the most to you in the past or ask a friend or pastor for guidance. Or perhaps you could ask God to reveal a new, deeper intimacy with you. Read the Psalms or other passages as though God were speaking personally to you.

Don't depend on your feelings to accurately reflect the truth. Depending on faith rather than feelings is like a pilot flying by instruments rather than sight. Pilots know that at times your senses tell you lies. You feel as if you're upright when you're upside down. You feel like you're flying straight when you're heading straight for the ground. Pilots have to learn to overcome those feelings and rely entirely on the instruments. Their survival depends on confidence in those instruments.

Illness is similar to flying in the clouds. You can't depend on your feelings. The Word is your instrument panel, accurately telling you what is true. God's Word says that you are incredibly valuable to him, beyond what you now know. He thinks of you several times a minute and is full of compassion toward you. "How precious to me are your thoughts, O God! How vast is the sum of them" (Ps. 139:17). "The Lord is righteous in all his ways and loving toward all he has made. The Lord is near to all who call on him, to all who call on him in truth" (Ps. 145:17–18). Don't let your feelings tell you otherwise.

WORK AT CONTROLLING YOUR ATTITUDE

While we don't always know why we suffer nor do we always have control over our circumstances, we can learn to have more control over our attitudes. Dr. Willhite tells the story of two elderly friends who had been stricken with severe arthritis early in their adult lives. One realized she had more time than others to pray and study God's Word. She became a very popular Sunday school teacher and a delight for others to be around. The other focused on her misery and grew bitter toward her family, friends, and eventually God. The first woman found joy; the second did not.[2] When you are suffering or fearful, looking for joy can seem impossible; there's no question it is a challenge. Others usually don't understand how hard it is. Don't ask them to. Simply fight to grab some joy, even just a little bit, because it will help you.

Cancer beckons you to focus on yourself. After all, you are suffering, and life is disrupted. You can certainly justify a little self-pity. But self-pity is destructive because it focuses your mind on your physical circumstances. As good as the short-term emotional gain feels, you should discard it for a better view of the Lord and his love. Expect to have to deliberately turn your mind to a God-ward focus. You may lapse into a self-focus and not even realize it. This is particularly true for prolonged suffering. I often see women battle the unseen enemy of self-pity, and I know it's easy to give in, give up, and quit resisting. But for those who persevere, the upbeat tempo of their approach to the challenges before them helps to fight cancer and its attending negative emotions. That's part of the reason I try to provide patients with a larger picture of what's happening to them—their battle isn't just about cancer, it's also about what they become spiritually as they wage the war.

Be willing to listen to those friends who try to pull you back to the positive. They might very well be God's messengers. Other friends might focus on your suffering.

Dr. Willhite found that the constant inquiries as to his well-being "weakened my focus on the Lord. Sadly, my prayers changed from 'Have Thine own way, Lord' to 'Lord, please remove that pain!'"[3] You may need to redirect friends to focus on the positive.

ACCEPT YOUR CIRCUMSTANCES

Accepting circumstances for what they are isn't the same as conceding victory to cancer. Accepting your weakness, your dependence on the Lord, and the possibility of unexpected circumstances are all signs of taking the first step toward true healing. With that battle won, your mind is free to move on to other aspects of life besides cancer. Not accepting that cancer is a part of your life acts like a tether, not letting your mind go. Paradoxically, with acceptance comes a severing of that tether.

Dr. Willhite writes, "When God allows us to suffer, it's not a detour; it's part of the main road. 'A man's steps are of the Lord. How then can a man understand his own way?' (Proverbs 20:24).

We may not know the reason for our suffering, but the Bible is very clear that suffering comes to accomplish God's purpose. As a sovereign and good God, He is not taken by surprise when His children suffer. His purposes are not thwarted, but they advance, through our suffering."[4]

Jacqueline, 54, found that cancer wasn't a detour for her either. "I was diagnosed with stage four lung cancer," she writes. "I was depressed and I despaired because the prognosis for my kind of cancer was six to nine months with chemotherapy. I started radiation and chemotherapy. Then I met a woman who lent me a book . . . that discussed the spiritual aspects of cancer. It said, 'There is a God who knows us and loves us, and God loves us even though God knows us.' The message was to believe in Him and pray, and He would ultimately answer our prayers whether it be in His time or our time. He has brought me an inner peace and tranquility I have never known in my entire life. He has filled a void in my life that was empty. I have accepted His Son, the Lord Jesus Christ, as my Redeemer and Savior. When people ask me whether I am angry or upset because I have cancer, I tell them no, because it has brought me to the Lord and Jesus Christ. Even if cancer takes my life, it will never take my soul."[5]

Do you know for certain that when this life is over, heaven will be your home? The Bible says you can have that assurance. First, admit to God that you sin and continually fall short of his standard of perfection (Rom. 3:23). Then acknowledge that Jesus, the perfect God-man, died in your place to bear the penalty (Rom. 5:8). The Bible says, "For God so loved the world that he gave his one and only Son, that whoever believes in him shall not perish but have eternal life" (John 3:16). How do you "believe in him"? Say a simple prayer telling the Father that you trust not in your own good works but in the works of his Son alone to open the way to an eternal life of intimacy with him.

COMFORT AND ENCOURAGE OTHERS

Often, after God has touched us in our agony and reminded us that he's doing something significant in the eternal scheme, he turns us around so we can offer others a loving shoulder. As Paul says, "Praise be to the God and Father of our Lord Jesus Christ, the Father of compassion and the God of all comfort, who comforts us in all our troubles, so that we can comfort those in any trouble with the comfort we ourselves have received from God" (2 Cor. 1:34).

We can provide comfort because we have a future hope. Pastor Danny Houze describes how he has seen this work.

A few years ago as Valerie Simonds was walking through her Dallas neighborhood, which is full of diverse, young professionals, she asked the Lord to somehow bring that community together in the fellowship of Christ. Valerie and her husband, Randy, a couple with four young children, have great vision not only for their church, of which I was the pastor, but also for their community.

And God answered her prayer in a way she and her family never would have fathomed. A little over two years ago doctors discovered a large mass in Val's brain that required immediate surgery. Family and friends gathered in the waiting room on the day of the procedure. All the dynamics that distinguish hospital waiting rooms were there: laughter, silence, prayer, and of course, questions about the future.

The outcome of the surgery was positive—most of the tumor was successfully removed. A small mass was left because of the risks involved in removing it. The doctors chose to use chemotherapy to deal with the remaining cancerous growth.

The last two years have been challenging for the Simonds family. Randy is an executive with an oil company that requires him to travel around the world, sometimes for weeks at a time. . . . Between Randy's travels, an active home, and the physical effects of chemo treatments, this young family has been stretched in all areas of their lives. Nonetheless they have responded with faith, dignity, and humor.

Not many weekends after a recent conversation they went through another series of turns on the roller-coaster ride that has marked their lives since the cancer was first detected. Val had just learned that the tumor had not grown, so she would not need to take chemo treatment for a while. This good news was followed by a weekend of small brain seizures. Her doctors told her that to combat the seizures she must now take strong anti-seizure medication. On top of this, the family's pet rabbit, Chloe, suddenly died. Val and Randy knew this was going to be hard on the kids, especially their youngest.

So that afternoon Val fixed herself a cup of tea and sat down to have a talk with her Lord. "Father," she said, "I have brain seizures and dead bunnies. What do You have to offer me?" God's response to her did not come with fireworks or visions but in a quiet whisper from His Word that has calmed her spirit and given her strength to continue to minister to her family: "Therefore we do not lose heart. Though outwardly we are wasting away, yet inwardly we are being renewed day by day. For our light and momentary troubles are achieving for us an eternal glory that far outweighs them all" (2 Cor. 4:16–17).

"I don't know why we fight against being weak," she said to me. "I am where I need to be in order to be used of Him."

The women in her neighborhood have united in fellowship, each rotating days of the week for fasting and prayer on her behalf. They have found themselves growing in their own faith. And so in her weakness Val is seeing her prayer answered as "an eternal weight of glory" far beyond what she would have ever imagined. And I, who was once her teacher, now find myself learning from my friend whose faith continues to shine brightly, even in the days of brain seizures and dead bunnies.[6]

God's purposes include instruction, but his reasons in allowing pain are often much broader than we might imagine. In Genesis we read that Joseph endured ill treatment, not only for character growth, but also because his circumstances would end up saving a nation. Sometimes difficulties provide an arena for God to bless all involved as well as for our growth. At the end of Job's struggle, he tells God, "My ears had heard of you but now my eyes have seen you" (Job 42:5).

Faith and Medical Treatment

Another common question for the patient and her family is how faith mixes with medicine. If you are trusting Jesus as your healer, how should you respond to a cancer diagnosis? Should you refuse all medical treatment, holding instead to complete trust in the Lord?

I would like to share some of my observations as a physician who loves Jesus dearly and also treats cancer patients. Jesus is our source of healing, but he might use doctors, nurses, and other health-care workers, or none of them, to do his work. However, if someone refuses medical treatment out of a desire to stand in faith, she may well be short-circuiting God's very provision for that circumstance. Following medical advice and trusting God are complementary, not conflicting, principles.

Jesus' severest critics couldn't refute his healings. The Pharisees worked diligently to find some grounds to discredit the Lord, and they stopped at nothing, including lying. Their anger, in an indirect way, verifies the authenticity of Jesus' healing. If they could have discredited the healing, their problem would have been solved. But they had to conclude that the only solution to their problem was to put the Lord to death.

Verification of authenticity is a consistent quality of true healing. The most brilliant physician in Jesus' day couldn't have cast doubt on the healing of the blind man (John 9) or any other healing Jesus did. So we know that Jesus is a healer. But how does he heal?

FAITH OBEYS

In all the Bible's miracles, including Jesus' healings, faith seems to be closely associated with obedience. When Jesus fed the five thousand (Matt. 14), the disciples, following Jesus' direction, distributed the food. Left to their own devices, they would have busied themselves looking for other solutions, checking out possible stores or other food sources. They already had suggested to Jesus that the way to feed the famished audience was to send them away to fend for themselves. Their words and behavior reveal that no one had in mind what the Lord was planning to do. It was Jesus' plan, and it was executed through obedience to his instructions.

When Moses parted the Red Sea and the children of Israel walked to the other side on dry ground, I would suggest that Moses in his wildest imagination couldn't have thought up such a thing. He had never seen anything like it, and it required of him a yielding and a level of obedience that is only cultivated with much practice. Moses stretched out his hand over the sea, then the Lord parted the waters (Ex. 14:21), not before. We call this "faith." It might also be called "obedience."

The miracles described in the Bible were conceived first by God and then executed through someone's obedience. Men and women made requests, but the answer was God's plan. When Peter stepped out of the boat and walked on water (Matt. 14), he requested permission, then stepped. When people came with requests to Jesus for healing, he answered differently every time. Perhaps this was not only because people are unique but also to keep us from devising a formula for healing. One consistent pattern does shine through each healing event: someone recognized Christ's authority and our dependence on God, yielded to God, and obeyed that authority. Again, that is what we call "faith."

The Bible also says several things that, in my mind, make it clear Jesus didn't stop healing when he ascended to heaven. I realize some children of God wouldn't agree that Jesus heals miraculously in current days, and I respect that opinion. But I maintain a different perspective. I believe his power actually is increased today, not diminished, when compared to biblical times. He said, "I tell you the truth, anyone who has faith in me will do what I have been doing. He will do even greater things than these, because I am going to the Father" (John 14:12).

EMPLOYING ADVISERS

So how do we cooperate with God today in receiving a miracle? Proverbs says that in an abundance of advisers is victory (Prov. 24:6). To me, the practical interpretation of that means that in areas where we have no expertise, we should seek out those with expertise or those who have studied that discipline. For instance, you wouldn't ask your accountant about tires for your car, nor would you ask an appliance salesperson for advice on legal matters. All truth—scientific, practical, or otherwise—is from God. He is the ultimate teacher, and knowledge is so vast that each of us can master only a small part of it.

Medical knowledge was given to humankind gradually over many centuries. The knowledge that physicians have comes from God. That doesn't mean inaccuracies don't exist. Medical knowledge is revised daily as we continue to learn more. But other, related professions that use different techniques than medical doctors aren't necessarily wrong. Our current understanding is imperfect, but those who pursue the truth eventually will arrive at similar conclusions.

When a Christian learns she has cancer, her response will reflect her understanding of God and how he works. Some will view physicians as instruments of God, trained to advise, counsel, and treat cancer. They will comply with the physician's recommendations out of a trust in God.

Others might see just the opposite. They view the physician as part of an impersonal, secular system that has no regard for God and that autonomously recommends whatever serves the medical establishment best. If that is the attitude, these people will turn away from a physician's recommendations and seek different answers from the Lord.

Still others view seeking help from medical science as the opposite of trusting God. They believe that to receive healing one must forgo medical treatment. Their intention is credible: They want to fight the good fight, to stand in faith, and to trust God against all odds. They see the physician as trying to destroy that faith rather than build it. To accept medical treatment is to give up on God and to abandon faith.

GOD'S PROVISION

Naaman's healing recorded in 2 Kings 5 offers enlightening insights into these issues. As commander of the Syrian army, Naaman was a dignitary in his society. However, he was a leper and desperate enough for healing that he lowered himself to go to his enemy, Israel, and seek out the prophet Elisha. Elisha sent word that Naaman was to wash himself in the Jordan seven times. This infuriated Naaman, both because he felt that he was important enough for a personal greeting from this lowly prophet and because the technique insulted his intelligence. It also gave honor to Israel's Jordan River rather than the rivers in his own country, which Naaman considered far superior. But his traveling companions convinced him to swallow his pride, and healing resulted.

What can we learn from Naaman's healing? Sometimes we think we know how God will work, when in fact he has chosen a different path. Our pride may get in the way of his plan, or we may fear what is recommended. God knew Naaman and knew what would cause Naaman to yield to God. God, not Naaman, would choose how Naaman would be healed. If Naaman had chosen his own ways, his healing would surely not have been realized. God is sovereign, and that's more important than our own pride or understanding.

Let's return to the Christian who considers forgoing medical treatment. What if God saw that person's need before the foundation of the earth? What if he prepared the physician years before this particular patient needed him or her, and brought their paths together by his sovereign will and plan? What if God is trying to speak to this patient through the physician's lips or to touch the patient through the physician's hands? It could be that to deny medical treatment is to short-circuit God's provision for this circumstance. Certainly Proverbs would agree with this thought when it suggests that wise decisions are reached as wise consultation is sought (24:6).

RECOGNIZE A HIGHER PURPOSE

Perhaps God is deepening our relationship with him and broadening our understanding of his ways. As much as God cares for our physical bodies, his higher purpose is to train our souls and prepare us for an eternal heritage. How he does that is beyond any of us to completely understand. Psalm 139:56 says that he has hemmed us in—behind and before—and laid his hand upon us. Such knowledge is too high and too wonderful; we cannot attain it. We may never comprehend what he is doing or why, but we can trust him.

When God works to develop our character, adverse circumstances seem to be a given. Joseph was sold into slavery (Gen. 37). David had to run for his life (1 Sam. 20). Moses was put out in the desert (Ex. 2). Job suffered physical loss and loss of health (Job 12).

God is the source of true healing, whether that means a physical cure in this life or being "promoted" to the next life. Jesus himself didn't presume upon God the Father when he was on the pinnacle of the temple during his temptation (Matt. 4). He could have thrown himself down, and the angels would have rescued him. But he chose not to test his Father. Stephen was stoned and died (Acts 7). Paul was stoned and lived (Acts 14:19). God holds our lives in his hand. Two individuals in similar circumstances find God chooses to act differently for each. True faith has confidence that God has our best interests in mind and that he will accomplish his purposes in his way.

John the Baptist was loved by Jesus, who described John this way: "Among those born of women there has not risen anyone greater than John the Baptist" (Matt. 11:11). John had prepared the way for Jesus. Yet even John didn't understand why Jesus left him in prison to be beheaded. Unsure if he had been mistaken about Jesus, John sent messengers to Jesus to ask, "Are you the one?" (Matt. 11:3). Jesus answered with compassion, "Blessed is the man who does not fall away on account of me" (v. 6). From John's perspective, Jesus had come to set the prisoner free, yet not John. One lesson we can take from this is that there is a plan that involves more than just this life, and we won't always understand God's ways. So it is with the woman who finds herself with breast cancer. Yes, God loves and cares for her. But his plan centers on a larger picture than the current events. Our job is to trust, to yield, to acknowledge his authority in our lives.

And through it all, remember that God is our source of healing. Following medical advice and trusting God are complementary, not conflicting, principles. See the hands of your doctors and nurses as those of the Lord ministering to you.

The spiritual journey through breast cancer is less tangible and often more difficult than the physical journey, but hopefully you've discovered some new ways to consider the spiritual side of cancer in this chapter.

The next section of the book, "The Medical Journey," will focus on the physical side of breast cancer, including what your medical options are, how to choose the right treatment for you, and what that treatment involves. I hope you'll carry into the reading of those chapters a sense that, through it all, the Great Physician is with you.

WHAT LOVED ONES CAN DO

Breast cancer affects the entire family and close friends. As each person respects the individual healing process for others, give time and space to one another. Space to struggle with questions before God. Space to be angry. Space to be unavailable at times. None of these things indicates unusual or abnormal behavior. What they do reflect is the process that the breast cancer patient and her loved ones go through. Be willing to say, "I need" or "I want" and listen carefully as others express their needs.

Be kind to everyone involved in this journey. Think of ways to help others along.

And help the cancer patient to focus on the spiritual journey she is taking. Help her to remember that cancer isn't just about the body; it's also about the soul. Don't try to offer easy or glib answers about what she is experiencing, for only she and God can understand that. Instead, think of ways to remind her that God is her companion on this journey. Pray aloud for her in her presence, read Scripture to her if she wishes. Let her know you are attentive to her spiritual needs.

PART 2

THE MEDICAL JOURNEY

CHAPTER 5

WHAT ARE YOUR SURGICAL OPTIONS?

With your medical and personal teams assembled, the next step in your journey through breast cancer is to choose among several treatment options. Once again, you are the one who makes the choices.

Most patients aren't used to having medical options when something goes wrong with their bodies; they expect to take their body to a doctor, who will fix it. But the medical world has developed a number of treatment possibilities for breast cancer. That gives you the opportunity to decide which road you'll travel toward health. You truly do have a strong say—the final say, actually—in your medical treatment. Enter into the experience with the knowledge that you are choosing the path you will take. That doesn't mean you should veer off the paths that are available, or that the path you do take won't be scary or have some big bumps in it. But it does mean that you aren't passive in this journey. And that's very good news.

The paths you have to consider at this point all involve a procedure that probably will sound pretty frightening to you, and that procedure is surgery. But, remember, this is a road to *recovery*, and that's a destination worth traveling this sort of road to get to.

In this chapter, I'm going to introduce you to your various surgical options. In the next chapter, I'll provide you with some advice on how to make the best decision. So we'll start out with understanding what the choices are; then we'll go about figuring out the best choice for you. As always, we'll hear from women who have traveled this road before you. They'll explain how they felt about the choices and which route they took.

Most of the time breast cancer surgery is done in two steps: a diagnostic procedure followed by a treatment procedure. We all have reason to be thankful that medicine has come to this point because, in the past, all breast cancer was treated with one surgery—a mastectomy. No decisions were required from the patient. A woman went into surgery not knowing whether she had cancer and found out in the recovery room based on the presence or absence of

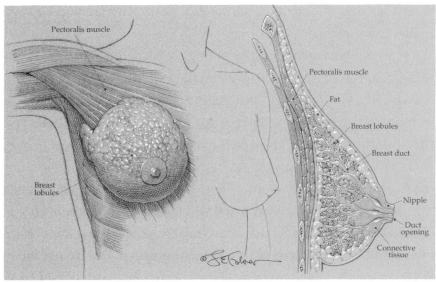

Pectoralis muscle

Pectoralis muscle

Fat

Breast lobules

Breast duct

Breast lobules

Nipple

Duct opening

Connective tissue

Lewis Calver

her breast. While this was quick, it also was traumatic. Now, with few exceptions, women have time to think and explore options before surgery is done.

Many of these options come as packages. So choosing one option would mean others automatically come with it. Sort of like choosing a vacation package: the airfare, hotel, and car rental are all part of the deal.

BREAST-CONSERVING THERAPY

With breast-conserving therapy, the choice to save as much of the breast as possible is made. This therapy consists of several steps, starting with a lumpectomy, which means the cancerous area in the breast is removed along with the normal-appearing breast tissue that surrounds the lump.

A pathologist examines this tissue and then issues a report within a few days. If the pathologist finds tumor cells at the edge of the tissue that was removed, called the "margins," additional breast tissue may need to be removed.

The second step of breast-conserving therapy is an axillary lymph node removal through an incision under the arm, different from the lumpectomy incision. This is a standard part of any breast cancer treatment.

Lymph nodes are small, bean-like structures found in groups throughout the body. They form part of the body's defense system against invaders such as bacteria and tumors. The nodes are removed from the underarm (axilla) because tumor cells from the breast may lodge there. Also, the removal of lymph nodes plays an important role in "staging" the tumor, or determining how advanced the cancer is. Be aware that because the lymph nodes are part of the body's defense system, once removed, the patient may be more susceptible to infection or swelling in that arm.

The third step for a woman electing to have breast-conserving therapy is usually chemotherapy, drugs administered intravenously to treat the entire body. We'll discuss the details of chemotherapy in an upcoming chapter. After chemotherapy, the patient receives daily radiation therapy for six to seven weeks. The radiation kills microscopic tumor cells, which could remain in the breast undetected.

Sometimes chemotherapy isn't required. If that's the case, the radiation starts when the surgeon establishes that the site operated on has healed, which usually is two or three weeks after surgery.

MASTECTOMY

Another alternative in the treatment of breast cancer is a mastectomy. Several types of mastectomy can be performed today.

RADICAL MASTECTOMY

Prior to the 1970s, radical mastectomy was the most commonly performed surgery. It involved removing not only the entire breast but also the muscle behind the breast and surrounding tissues. Today this procedure is used only when the pectoralis muscle, the muscle behind the breast, is involved with tumor growth, which is rare.

TOTAL OR SIMPLE MASTECTOMY

A total mastectomy (also called a simple mastectomy) removes all the breast tissue but not the lymph nodes. This is done most commonly for noninvasive cancer (tumor cells inside the ducts or lobules in the breast that have not spread outside the ducts) or as a preventive measure because of a patient's high risk of developing breast cancer.

MODIFIED RADICAL MASTECTOMY

Modified radical mastectomy is currently done for invasive cancer (tumor cells that have spread outside the original duct system into surrounding breast tissue). This procedure involves removing all the breast tissue and some of the lymph nodes under the arm without removing muscle. This means the arm normally retains the same strength as before surgery.

Because a mastectomy removes all the breast tissue that could harbor tumor cells, radiation therapy usually isn't necessary. But radiation is needed after a mastectomy if, for example, tumors are over two inches in size, tumors are attached to the chest muscle, or four or more lymph nodes contain tumor cells. These are situations in which there is a concern that tumor cells could still be present on the remaining chest wall or underarm area.

SENTINEL NODE BIOPSY

Part of the surgical procedure involves the lymph nodes and exploring whether cancer has moved to this area. For breast cancer, like many other cancers, the most important predictor of how aggressive a tumor will behave is linked to whether tumor cells are detected in the lymph nodes.

For many years the normal procedure for treating breast cancer was to remove all the underarm lymph nodes. Because lymph nodes are found throughout the body, other nodes nearby take over the work of the ones removed. In recent years, breast cancer often has been detected early, before tumor cells have reached the lymph nodes. That has prompted research in better ways to find and remove only the lymph nodes most likely to contain tumor cells.

Researchers have found that the spread of cancer cells to the lymph nodes under the arm usually occurs in an orderly fashion, which is why the first affected node or two are called the "sentinel lymph nodes." This has led to the sentinel node biopsy in which the tumor site in the breast is injected prior to surgery with a radioactive tracer or a blue dye or both. These migrate to the lymph nodes, allowing the surgeon to identity one or two nodes that are first in the drainage pathway from the tumor area. The dye doesn't indicate whether tumor cells are present in these nodes, but rather shows which lymph nodes to examine first. If those nodes are clear of tumor cells, then additional lymph nodes might not be removed. If the sentinel nodes contain tumor cells, the surgeon will recommend the removal of the remainder of the lymph nodes to avoid leaving tumor cells behind.

AXILLARY DISSECTION

Every woman has a unique number of lymph nodes, but normally about twenty or more nodes are removed with a complete axillary (underarm) dissection. Women who have all the nodes removed are more susceptible to swelling or infection in the arm and need to take precautions to prevent this, which we'll discuss in chapter 13. These complications can occur soon after surgery or

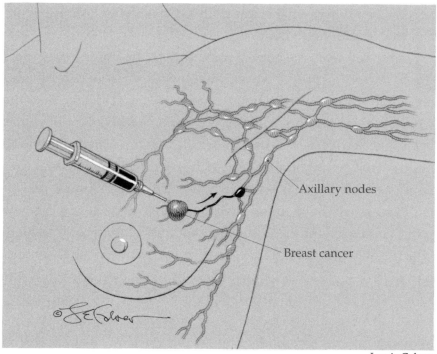

Lewis Calver

many years later. There may be some permanent numbness under the arm extending to the upper inner arm.

Now, before moving on, let's take a collective deep breath and summarize the surgical options.

- **Lumpectomy:** Removal of a limited area of breast tissue that includes the cancer and surrounding tissue. This has also been called tylectomy, quadrantectomy (which removes a fourth of breast tissue), segmental resection, or partial mastectomy.
- **Total mastectomy:** Removal of the complete breast without removing the lymph node area under the arm. Breast tissue often extends into the axilla (underarm) where lymph nodes are located, and one or two nodes may be removed in order to remove all breast tissue.
- **Modified radical mastectomy:** Removal of the complete breast and some of the lymph nodes under the arm.
- **Axillary dissection:** Removal of lymph nodes under the arm. This is through a separate incision when a lumpectomy or skin-sparing mastectomy is done.
- **Sentinel node biopsy:** Removal of the first lymph nodes under the arm in the drainage pathway from the cancerous area in the breast.

Twenty-five-year-old Tonya, whom you met in chapter 1, had a modified radical mastectomy. "My cancer was fast-growing," she said. "But only two of eleven lymph nodes were involved."

Patti chose a mastectomy partly because her husband lost his first wife to breast cancer when it recurred after five years. Both Patti and her husband felt that a mastectomy was preferable to avoid worrying about the breast. "I wanted as much removed as possible," Patti said. "And then I cried when I told the doctor; I knew it was the right choice, but it still was hard."

RECONSTRUCTION

Another choice that you make after a mastectomy is whether to pursue breast reconstruction or wear a prosthesis (artificial breast). Reconstruction may be done with the initial mastectomy or months or years later.

Reconstruction affects how the woman sees herself but usually has little bearing on how others see her. A woman may think she is doing it for her husband or significant other, but that partner in most cases feels the same about her with or without a reconstructed breast.

Reconstruction can make a difference, however, in how the woman feels about her body and its attractiveness, which can significantly affect her quality of life. Some do reconstruction so that wearing a swimsuit or low neckline is less of a problem. Others feel better about themselves with both breasts. Some turn down reconstruction because of the additional surgery and recovery time. After becoming informed about what is involved, you are the one to make the decision. Neither your cancer surgeon nor your partner can make that choice for you.

If you choose to reconstruct at the time of the initial surgery, the surgeon will perform a skin-sparing mastectomy, removing breast tissue and lymph nodes but leaving most of the skin envelope. The areola (darker pigmented skin around the nipple) and skin directly overlying the cancer area in the breast is removed, but much of the rest of the skin is left in place. Your cancer surgeon will complete the mastectomy, and the plastic surgeon will then do the reconstruction.

Because of coordinating two surgeons' schedules, this may delay the operation a few days. That shouldn't make a difference in your outcome—although waiting can make you anxious.

Reconstruction at the time of the mastectomy has the advantage that you come out of surgery with the main part of the reconstruction completed, which prevents another hospitalization a few months later. The surgery might last several hours or most of the day, depending on the type of reconstruction. Often, short surgeries may be done later to finish some of the details such as nipple reconstruction. The immediate reconstruction has become the most popular alternative for women electing to go this route.

Don't feel you have to do reconstruction immediately if you are not certain that you want reconstruction or feel overwhelmed by the additional decisions this entails. You can always make that choice months or years later.

Not all women are candidates for immediate reconstruction. If radiation therapy is needed after a mastectomy, reconstruction is delayed for several months after radiation is completed to create the most optimal conditions for a good cosmetic result.

Women planning to have chemotherapy can have immediate reconstruction. Chemotherapy can start at about the same time it would without reconstruction, with a delay of only a week or two in some cases to allow for healing.

Dee chose reconstructive surgery after a lot of thought—nearly a full year's worth. She didn't want reconstruction initially but later opted for it. "As an active female, who spent a lot of time outdoors in the sun, I found the silicone breast to be uncomfortably hot," she explained. "My son played a lot of sports; so many times I would be at a ball game in temperatures of 100 degrees. It wouldn't be long before my shirt was damp from the sweat running down from under my bra. On one occasion I took my prosthesis out and put it in a friend's ice chest. In the excitement of the game, I forgot about it. On my ride home, I laughingly asked my husband, 'Honey, can we turn around? I forgot something.' My daughter smiled up at me—this was the second time I had left my breast behind! That day I decided that, if I couldn't keep track of it, I needed a permanent one I was comfortable with at all times."

Twelve years after the reconstruction Dee says, "In all honesty, I don't remember what my old breast was like. To me, the reconstructive breast is my 'natural' breast. I love the way God created our memory to help us make adjustments. We soon forget the pain of childbirth, morning sickness, twisted ankles, the flu. That's the way I feel about my cancer. The surgery and chemotherapy are long forgotten. The new breast is now part of me."

Jyme, pronounced "Jimmie," 48, laughs on recounting her first encounter with a plastic surgeon. She was still trying to absorb the news that she had breast cancer and had never dreamed of altering her A-cup breasts. She had a thousand pinecones in her stomach when she went to see a plastic surgeon with her husband, Steve, and close friends Vicki and Hal.

"We were all in the examining room when in walked 'Renaissance Man' surgeon wearing European clogs," Jyme recalls. "He explained various types of reconstruction and what he planned to do and then motioned us toward his portfolio of women's breasts. Apparently he thought we would like to pick out a pair."

Jyme sat there in shock. "But my husband and my friend leaped from their chairs and raced over to look at the portfolio. Then they proceeded to discuss the 'best set' for me. As I sat with mouth agape, my husband of a quarter century and my closest friend were picking out my new breasts—and it didn't take long. Immediately they pointed to a 'pair' in the portfolio." Her loved ones' lighthearted approach shifted the mood for Jyme and made something fun out of an otherwise tense afternoon.

Before Jody met with a variety of physicians to consider her options, she was leaning toward a mastectomy and reconstruction. But then she concluded, "After visiting the plastic surgeon and listening to what he would do to reconstruct my left breast, I realized it was going to be a difficult surgery. A mastectomy in itself is also more difficult to recover from than a lumpectomy, even if, as in my case, they will take a whole segment during the lumpectomy." Jody opted for a lumpectomy. But she did so after weighing her options and understanding what was involved with each choice.

Reconstruction usually isn't done after a lumpectomy. Some institutions are researching that possibility for women who have a large area of the breast removed, but filling a partial defect and attaining a good, long-term cosmetic result is difficult to do.

If you do not elect to do reconstruction, you will wear an artificial prosthesis after mastectomy. Partial prostheses may also be used in some cases after lumpectomy to help with symmetry. Breast prostheses are designed to look natural and have the approximate weight of the opposite breast.

Josefa, who chose to go with what she calls "false breasts," took her husband with her to order her prostheses. "It surprised me when one of the employees told him, 'Sir, congratulations, you are a wonderful husband. This is the first time I've seen a husband with his wife in this store.'" Josefa found her husband's support through the entire breast cancer journey a strong source of encouragement and strength.

Another woman relates how humor can help to keep one in the swim of things. One day she went swimming with her friends. "My cute two-piece swimsuit was designed to hold my prosthesis in place, or so I thought," she recounted. "After a rather graceful dive, I climbed out of the pool and stretched on my lounge chair. My girlfriends started to smile, and one asked, 'I wonder if silicone floats?' Before I could process that comment, my friends were looking into the pool. Several seconds passed before I realized they were looking for my breast in the water. We all laughed as we walked around the edge. Now it was a game—who could find the breast first? Soon we all spotted my 'C' cup resting on the drain. We laughed about that for days, and I am sure my awesome friends will tell that story for years to come."

Brenda, 38, who had an early-stage cancer, was faced with these choices. Her decision was immediate. "I had a friend who had had a lumpectomy, and the cancer came back; so I opted for a mastectomy with an immediate reconstruction."

Brenda made her choice by comparing her situation to her friend's. But the friend's recurrence in no way indicated that Brenda would also have a recurrence. It did mean that, for Brenda, anxiety about the cancer returning might outweigh saving her breast.

Tonya, Jody, and Brenda all made different choices for different reasons. And, while many of the factors that are weighed are the same for everyone facing breast cancer, those factors weigh different amounts for each person.

Now that you understand more what your choices are, in the next chapter, we'll work through those factors to help you reach your decision.

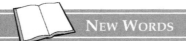

NEW WORDS

In situ: Cancer inside the duct system that has not yet broken through the duct wall to invade the surrounding tissues.

Invasive, or infiltrating, duct cancer: The most common type of breast cancer, originating in the duct system in the breast.

Lymph nodes: Bean-like structures that are found all over the body. They are often found in clusters, or grouped together, and function like filters to protect the body from bacteria, cancer cells, and other foreign substances.

Prosthesis: An artificial breast made from silicone or synthetic materials designed to be about the same weight as the natural breast.

Staging: A system of cancer classification from stage 1, the earliest breast cancers, to stage 4, advanced breast cancer. The system is designed to help with treatment decisions and prognosis.

STRENGTHENING THOUGHTS
FROM GOD'S WORD

"In all your ways acknowledge him, and he will make your paths straight" (Prov. 3:6).

"May the Lord direct your hearts into God's love and Christ's perseverance" (2 Thess. 3:5).

CHAPTER 6

CHOOSING THE RIGHT SURGERY FOR YOU

From the time of the initial diagnosis, I've found many women are impatient to move on to the next step. They fear that waiting to really think about their options can jeopardize the outcome. Let me assure you, if surgery is completed within about a month, the outcome will not change. Give yourself time to think, ask questions, explore, and perhaps get several opinions.

But realize, too, that once you've determined which procedure you want, getting it done brings immense relief. That certainly was true for Jane.

At age 44, Jane found that once she started to work with a surgeon, events unfolded rapidly. "I saw the surgeon on Monday, and she could fit in a surgery on Thursday. She was leaving for an international trip on Friday afternoon. So on Thursday morning she removed the lump and sent it for biopsy. Malignant. By noon she had told us, and we had the choice of more surgery the next morning to remove lymph nodes and either clean up the margins or do a mastectomy. If we didn't have surgery then, we'd need to wait two weeks till her return."

Jane and her husband opted for surgery the next morning. Suddenly they were facing pre-op, scheduling, blood tests, X-rays, and racing home to process it all, tell their children, and decide on the type of surgery.

"Through tears and prayers, I decided on the mastectomy," Jane said, "because that was where I felt God's peace."

What are the factors that help to determine whether a woman should have a lumpectomy or a mastectomy? Follow-up data after many years have shown that both a lumpectomy with radiation therapy and a mastectomy yield good results, that one isn't necessarily "safer" than the other.

When faced with this decision, you may feel that your doctor has turned you out on an ice rink expecting you to glide gracefully even though you've never skated. In fact, the physician knows this is new and stressful for you, and he or she is available to help and guide you. Your doctor wants to see you healthy and happy as much as you want to get through this and back to familiar ground.

So why does a patient have to make these choices at such a stressful time? Why not do a lumpectomy every time and spare the woman the anxiety of making a decision she might feel incapable of? Several factors need to be considered in making the right choice for you, but only you can examine these factors and make a choice.

Factors to consider in deciding on the best surgical option:
1. Personal preferences
2. Characteristics of the tumor
3. Size of the breast in relation to the size and location of the tumor

---

> 4. Medical factors other than breast cancer
>
> 5. Logistics

PERSONAL PREFERENCES

Let's consider personal factors first. Two patients with exactly the same circumstances—the same size tumor in exactly the same place in the same breast—might make different choices for personal reasons. One woman might be young with several relatives, including her mother, who had breast cancer. Once she develops breast cancer, her priority is to remove all breast tissue not only because of her current tumor but also because of her concern about breast cancer occurring again in either breast. She chooses a mastectomy and reconstruction because for her it relieves anxiety.

Another woman with exactly the same circumstances might have seen her mother struggle emotionally after a mastectomy years ago or been traumatized herself by a close relative's surgery and decided a mastectomy would be her last resort. To her, lumpectomy is a much more attractive choice.

What personal factors are on your mind?

PATHOLOGY

A tumor, when examined with a microscope by a pathologist, has a characteristic appearance. A pathologist generally can determine the originating tissue for a tumor based on those characteristics. For example, a tumor from the colon will look different from a tumor from the breast. That's how the pathologist can be certain that a tumor started in the breast and didn't spread there from somewhere else. Some tumors have such abnormal-looking cells that the originating tissue can't be determined, but that isn't a typical situation.

Cancers that form a single lump in the breast and can be removed completely with clear margins (no cancer is found in the edges of the tissue removed) are best suited for a lumpectomy. But cancer cells sometimes grow in several areas in the breast (which is called "multifocal" or "multicentric" disease). When that's the case, the patient may be better served with a mastectomy. For the recurrence rate to be low after a lumpectomy, all cancer cells along with a margin of surrounding normal breast tissue must be removed.

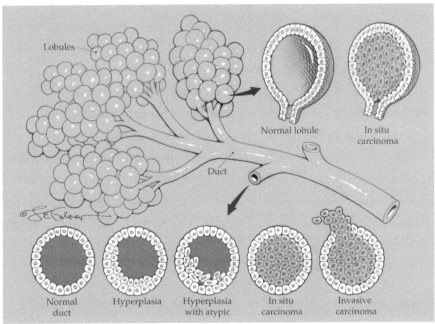

Lewis Calver

Different types of breast cancer have different characteristics. The most common types include the following:

INVASIVE, OR INFILTRATING, DUCT CANCER

Typically shows up as a lump a woman feels in her breast or is seen as a mass on a mammogram. About 70 percent of breast cancer consists of this type. Its name comes from the belief that it originates in the breast's duct system, the branching network of channels that carry milk to the nipple.

Cindy's path to her diagnosis was somewhat unusual. She had a rib that occasionally slipped out of place and caused pain in her right breast. After a flare-up that kept her in pain for three weeks, she visited her chiropractor for treatment. At the same time, she felt a soreness and a fatty thickening of tissue in that breast. "I did nothing for two weeks," she recalls. "Then I told my husband, who said to get a mammogram." A week later, Cindy had a mammogram, then a sonogram, and then a needle biopsy. The diagnosis: breast cancer.

INTRADUCTAL BREAST CANCER

This is also called DCIS ("duct carcinoma in situ") or "in situ breast cancer." Thought to be the preinvasive form of infiltrating duct cancer, it's often found adjacent to infiltrating duct breast cancer. The term means that the tumor cells are all inside the breast ductal system and haven't broken through a duct wall to invade surrounding breast tissue where they have access to the lymph nodes and blood vessels draining the breast.

Before that invasion occurs, a woman usually is unable to feel the intraductal carcinoma. It hasn't yet caused a lump and usually is detected by a change on a mammogram. Once it breaks through the duct wall and becomes invasive, it causes a hardening, or a lump, in the surrounding tissues that you can feel.

Until mammograms were commonly done, DCIS was rarely detected. Only about 2 percent of women detected breast cancer at this stage, and those were mostly palpable lumps. Now that patients commonly have screening mammograms, 12 to 15 percent of breast cancer is detected at the in situ stage.[1]

When breast cancer is found while it is in situ (inside the duct), the prognosis is excellent. If adequately treated, 98 percent of women will make a complete recovery with little possibility of recurrence outside the breast. But intraductal cancer sometimes is diffuse in the ductal system of the breast. Even if it's detected because of abnormal calcifications on a mammogram, the tumor area can go beyond the calcifications and be larger than it appears on the mammogram. For that reason, although DCIS is considered the earliest stage of breast cancer, a lumpectomy may be impossible. If the tumors are too spread out in the breast, they can be treated with a mastectomy, often with a reconstruction at the same time.

When DCIS is spread over a large area in the breast, it doesn't mean the prognosis is worse as long as the pathologist sees no invasive breast cancer. It's just an odd fact that some early breast cancers found on a mammogram can't be treated with a lumpectomy.

INVASIVE, OR INFILTRATING, LOBULAR CARCINOMA

This cancer is less common, making up about 20 percent of breast cancers. Because it was thought to originate in breast lobules, those tiny, saclike structures that create the breast's milk, it was given its name. This cancer looks different under the microscope than infiltrating duct cancer and behaves differently, making it difficult to detect either through a physical exam or a mammogram until the tumor is quite large. At times it forms an obvious lump just like ductal carcinoma, but other times it sends tiny strands, or fingers, of tumor cells around normal structures in the breast.

This tumor may be challenging to excise by lumpectomy because of the difficulty in detecting the extent of the tumor. If discovered when it's small and the margins (edges of the tissue removed by the surgeon) around the tumor are clear of tumor cells, the patient does as well with a lumpectomy as patients with infiltrating duct cancer do. Over a twenty-year follow-up, slightly more women with invasive *lobular* cancer develop a new cancer in the opposite breast (20 percent) compared to invasive *duct* cancer (15 percent).

LOBULAR CARCINOMA IN SITU

Also called LCIS or "lobular neoplasia," the cancer was given this name in the 1940s, when medical researchers thought it represented a malignancy. Although it was reclassified as premalignant long ago, the name stuck and can cause anxiety when a patient is told she has lobular carcinoma in situ. This cancer doesn't make a lump in the breast and doesn't show up on a mammogram. It's usually found when breast tissue is removed for another reason.

Of the women who have LCIS discovered on their biopsy, around 20 percent will develop cancer over the next twenty years. The biopsy's location doesn't indicate which breast will develop cancer, or if it will happen at all. Most of the time women with this finding elect to do careful follow-up, but no further surgery. Thus, LCIS is considered a risk factor for breast cancer, but not actually cancer.

OTHER CANCER TYPES

A number of other less common tumors can occur in the breast, such as tubular carcinoma and medullary carcinoma. Some of these tumors actually are less aggressive than the more common infiltrating duct cancer. The treatment options are similar to those for infiltrating duct cancer.

Be aware of the findings in your pathology report; that report will be an important factor in deciding which direction you should take for your treatment. Also, understanding the likelihood of recurrence for your type of breast cancer will help in your decision-making.

BREAST SIZE

Another factor that can influence the decision to have a lumpectomy or a mastectomy is the breast's size relative to the tumor's size. Women with small breasts may have a significant defect if even a small tumor is excised, while women with larger breasts may have a large area removed and still have an acceptable cosmetic result.

Women wanting a lumpectomy and requiring removal of a large part of the breast have several options. Completing a few weeks of chemotherapy prior to surgery may decrease the tumor size enough to allow for a lumpectomy with good cosmetic results. The timing of chemotherapy either before or after surgery hasn't been found to affect long-term recovery, but doing it prior to surgery may enable some women to opt for a lumpectomy who otherwise wouldn't be able to.

Large-breasted women might have difficulty with a lumpectomy because of the significant volume of tissue requiring radiation. Consultation with a radiation oncologist prior to surgery can clear up any questions. Radiation therapy after a lumpectomy in some cases causes permanent swelling in the breast, and large-breasted women seem to be more susceptible to this. So, if a woman already experiences shoulder pain because of the weight of her breasts, that condition could worsen after she completes radiation. Breast reduction can be done after a lumpectomy, but it could make follow-up of the lumpectomy area more difficult. Some women who have had shoulder or back problems with large breasts opt for a mastectomy, reconstruction, and a reduction of the opposite breast.

Cancers directly under the nipple were once thought not to be amenable to lumpectomy because they require removal of the nipple itself. Many women now choose to have a lumpectomy and have the nipple reconstructed after they have finished all of their cancer treatment.

Women with breast implants may develop much harder breasts after the radiation therapy needed for a lumpectomy. This is called "capsular contracture" and is the body's normal response to the implant, but the effect is exaggerated after radiation therapy.

OTHER MEDICAL CONDITIONS

Other medical conditions may play a role in the decision for breast conservation. Women who have collagen vascular disease—a class of diseases to which rheumatoid arthritis, scleroderma, and lupus belong—might not tolerate radiation. Their normal tissues show a tendency to overreact to the radiation therapy, and that can lead to painful scarring and hardening of the breast.

Women who have already had chest radiation therapy might not tolerate more radiation therapy, eliminating a lumpectomy as an option. Normal tissue can handle only a certain amount of radiation; one area of the body can typically have radiation therapy only once. By the way, the energy and dose of radiation used to kill tumor cells is much higher than that used for diagnostic X-rays. So previous X-rays (even numerous X-rays) will not alter the ability to have radiation therapy for cancer.

Pregnancy is another factor that may influence the decision about surgery. Many pregnant patients can have a lumpectomy, with delay of radiation therapy until after delivery.

What medical factors might effect your decision?

FAMILY HISTORY

Patients that have several first-degree (mother, sisters, daughters) or second-degree (aunts, cousins) relatives who have had breast cancer might take into consideration their family history when choosing between a lumpectomy or a mastectomy. Genetic counseling often is available at major cancer centers to help you sort through the issues and to decide whether to have genetic testing. But the counseling and testing can take several months, which might delay your treatment longer than is wise to wait.

Some women whose families have a significant history of breast cancer choose to have a prophylactic mastectomy. This total mastectomy is done when no cancer has been diagnosed to prevent a possible occurrence. Reconstruction usually is done immediately after this surgery. While a prophylactic mastectomy substantially reduces the risk of breast cancer, it's not a guarantee. A few breast lobules could be left behind with the remaining skin.

LOGISTICS

Some women opt for a mastectomy because they live outside of a metropolitan area and daily transportation to and from radiation therapy would be burdensome. If that's your situation, you might be able to stay with friends or relatives closer to an appropriate facility. Ask around; you might be surprised at the possibilities.

DECISION TIME

In determining which procedure you will choose, you and your family need to feel free to ask the surgeon questions—even if the material has been covered previously, perhaps even several times. A win-win situation is when a patient understands the treatment being recommended and the reasons for it.

As I've said earlier, you also need to feel free to obtain a second opinion. This is a healthy educational experience and helps to solidify your understanding of the treatment options.

The following questions are important for you to ask your surgeon to help you make the most knowledgeable decision possible:

- How long will the surgery last?
- Where will the incision be? What will it look like? Will I have stitches?
- When will I get the pathology report?
- How long will I be in the hospital?
- What kind of help will I need at home?

- Will I have to change a bandage or have drains at home? Who will teach me about those things?
- How long will I be home before going back to work or resuming normal responsibilities?
- When can I drive?
- When can I resume my diet, exercise class, get my nails done?
- What special exercises or care will my surgery arm need?

Put yourself two years down the road from this situation. Choose the surgical option that you believe will serve you best long term. Although a mastectomy and reconstruction require a longer recovery period than a lumpectomy, within several months your treatment will be complete. Don't let the specifics of the short-term drive your decision. Consider who you are as a whole and decide with the longer view in mind.

Deb shares how she felt after making her decision to have surgery. "I quickly scheduled the date. I was mentally ready. I was nervous, of course, and lost some sleep, but I think that was fairly normal. One night I wrote out a 'to do' list of things I felt I needed to do if I had less than a year to live. A few nights later, I tore the list up and wrote a new list, this time titled 'Things not to worry about.' I only wrote one word—'tomorrow.'"

PREPARING FOR SURGERY

Knowing your surgery is just around the corner, you'll find anxiety will be one of your biggest challenges. Here are some tips that Deb employed to help her deal with the waiting time.

"In the days before surgery, I focused on lighthearted activities. I had a manicure, went for walks, read a romance novel. I certainly knew enough about breast cancer already, so I shelved those books.

A few times every day I would stop to relax, breathe deeply, and clear my mind. These activities helped to reduce the stress of waiting, but the real peace came from another source.

"My relationship with Jesus had been touch-and-go for years. I had always prayed a lot, but now that wasn't enough. I found that, with this huge event threatening to change my life, I needed to recommit to God. His presence was always there, but I needed to find a way to strengthen my conviction and my belief. To believe with all my heart, and to trust, and accept that he was in control. With him I could do this cancer thing with less worry.

"So along with my romance novel, I bought my first devotional. I knew my power was in him and in his Word. I never had spent long periods of time learning from the Bible. I knew Jesus as my Savior, I trusted the cross, now I needed to live the Resurrection—enjoy the relationship I could have with him. It was a refreshing time."

Before your surgery date, think about what information you want your surgeon or family members to communicate. If your spouse plans to make calls after your surgery, think about whom you do and don't want him to communicate with. For instance, if you have an ill parent, would it be better to call that person right away to relieve concern, or do you plan to wait until you are back on your feet to share medical information? Plan for someone close to you to communicate with extended family and friends rather than ask your surgeon to call someone who was unable to be at the hospital.

Know the anticipated time in surgery and how many days you'll be in the hospital. As surgical and anesthesia techniques have improved, shorter hospitals stays are the norm. In general, I've found that patients rest better, eat better, and recover faster at home rather than in the hospital, which tends to encourage staying in bed.

Ask where the incision will be and whether you will have stitches or staples afterwards. Know about any drains, who will care for them, and when instruction will take place.

Understanding these details will help you to feel that you are part of the process and won't be caught off guard by a detail for which information was readily available before surgery, but you didn't realize you should ask about it.

Should family stay the night at the hospital? Think this through ahead of time. Balance the need for them to get rest versus their sense of responsibility for you and what you might need, especially in the first twenty-four hours when you won't be as alert mentally as you normally are. This may be an opportunity to suggest extended family members, such as parents or siblings, stay with you. Often they want to be involved and feel they are a part of the process.

THE DAY OF SURGERY

Don't expect a lot of new information the day of your surgery. The immediate goal is to recover physically. The breast tissue and lymph nodes that are removed will be carefully evaluated, and a report will be available several days after the surgery.

But do give yourself room to have an emotional response to the surgery. Sandy wrote in her journal about the loss of her breasts. "I know, I know, I'm more than my breasts, but I'm grieving this beautiful part of me that ended up in a bowl. This is a huge loss. Very wise friends have advised me not to play down or ignore this loss."

Deb's surgery caused her minimal pain. "I followed my doctor's instructions by stretching my arm above my head starting the day after surgery. I never babied the surgery site."

For Deb, the painful part was waiting for the pathology report. Her experience as a nurse helped, though. Her advice to patients is to call your surgeon if you haven't heard the results on the day promised. "Surgeons are very busy and see lots of reports daily. Some days they may not even go to the office because they've been in surgery all day. I know they care about each patient, but I think often they don't realize the stress that occurs waiting for that report. Talk to their nurse and leave all the phone numbers where you can be reached. The nurse should always be your advocate to help meet your needs."

RECOVERY FROM SURGERY

Kelly's recuperation was remarkable. "I had surgery on Monday and was released Tuesday afternoon. My husband and I went to the movies on the way home and saw *Monsters, Inc.*" Now, I can't promise you that you'll be ready to go to the movies the day after your surgery, but Kelly's experience can provide a bit of perspective on how well the surgery can go. Each woman's experience is as unique as she is.

After either a lumpectomy or a mastectomy, the arm tends to stiffen and may hurt when moved. Typically these symptoms are most noticeable after two or three weeks. Specific exercises help you to regain your range of motion in the affected arm. Your surgeon will guide you as to when you should start these. Stretching and exercising the arm for many weeks and even months following surgery is important; the exercises markedly decrease the pain, and mobility should return rapidly. If not, you may be referred to a physical therapist for help.

Numbness in your underarm and on the back of your arm close to the armpit is common. The nerve that carries sensation to that area is removed with the lymph nodes. Such numbness is often permanent. If you are painfully sensitive in the area, gentle rubbing of the skin will help. The pain lessens and resolves itself within a few weeks after the surgery.

A cordlike structure can develop down the inside surface of the arm, extending to your elbow or below. This is a normal part of the healing and will resolve without any special treatment within a few months after surgery. The exact cause isn't known, but it's possible a lymphatic vessel is scarring down. But it is uncomfortable and can cause diminished shoulder mobility. Proper exercising helps with the pain and in retaining mobility.

Find a way to stay physically active after surgery. You will have some fatigue and won't be able to keep up with your previous schedule right away, but the more active you stay, the faster you recover. Being physically active also will help you to focus on subjects other than the surgery.

Before your surgery or after, listen to tapes or CDs that relax and soothe. Some women don't want to use music they enjoy because they don't want to associate it with cancer.

BREAST CANCER STAGING

Several tests help to determine how likely breast cancer cells are to spread outside the breast. These tests will be done either prior to surgery or right after and are called "staging" because the cancer's stage of growth is classified by a number on a scale from 0 to 4.

If breast cancer moves into the blood or lymphatic channels, it tends to show up next in the bones, lungs, or liver. Those areas are checked with a chest X-ray, blood tests, bone scan or survey, and a liver sonogram or CT scan. Most of these tests are done prior to surgery, but can be done either before or after the operation.

Any symptoms a patient might have also could result in tests appropriate for that symptom. Each physician has a preference as to which tests are used and how frequently each is done. But the tests can pick up only tumors a fourth of an inch or greater in size, which means the tumor already contains millions of cells. Nothing at this time can determine if one or two cells have migrated out of the breast, which is why additional treatment such as chemotherapy or hormonal therapy often follows surgery. These treatments are focused on eradicating those cells if present.

BONE SCAN

A bone scan involves injecting a radioactive substance into a vein. This substance migrates to the bones and is scanned a couple of hours later. The radiologist is looking for "hot" spots: areas where the bone is more active. Arthritis, a recent fracture or other irritation, or perhaps infection can cause hot spots. The hot areas are then X-rayed, which usually will show whether the area is active because of tumor cells or some other cause. Some physicians may do a skeletal survey, which is a series of X-rays that give information equivalent to the bone scan.

LIVER SONOGRAM OR CT

A liver sonogram or a CT scan evaluates the liver and abdomen. The sonogram uses sound waves with no radiation involved. The CT scan uses radiation. Both tests give different kinds of information, so both may be used in some cases.

Doctors vary on how many of these preliminary tests should be done if an individual has early breast cancer since the tests usually come back negative. Most physicians agree the tests are worth doing after the initial diagnosis, and repeated only if new symptoms occur. The tests aren't repeated each year because they don't detect a recurrence (metastasis) any earlier than can be found with a history and physical exam by a cancer doctor.

THE STAGES

After surgery and the above tests have been completed, the breast cancer is staged. This general classification helps physicians determine further treatment and the prognosis.

Stage 0 is intraductal carcinoma, or DCIS. The tumor hasn't become invasive and is unlikely to have spread outside the breast. A woman has an excellent prognosis with stage 0 disease.

Stage 1 is an invasive tumor 2 cm (just under an inch) or less in size with no lymph node involvement.

Stage 2 is an invasive tumor 2 to 5 cm in size or with lymph node involvement.

Stage 3 is an invasive tumor more than 5 cm in size with lymph nodes involved that may have other features physicians consider locally advanced cancer (skin or chest wall involvement).

Stage 4 is cancer that has spread outside the breast to other organs, called "metastatic disease." When a woman has breast cancer and later has cancer in her bones, that usually means the breast cancer spread to the bones, that is, metastasized to the bones. Breast cancer also can spread to other organs, such as the lungs and liver.

ESTROGEN AND PROGESTERONE RECEPTORS

In addition to staging, the pathology report contains information on other factors that play a role in determining how aggressive the tumor is. One of these is the tumor's estrogen and progesterone receptor status. Normal breast tissue cells have receptors for both of these female hormones. These receptors cause normal breast tissue to grow and mature properly. When a cell becomes cancerous, it may retain some of the characteristics of a normal breast tissue cell, such as the receptors, or it may lose them. When the receptors are retained on the cancerous cells, a hormone blocker may be used as a part of the treatment. I'll discuss this in chapter 7.

MARKERS

Other factors that help to determine a tumor's aggressiveness include its growth rate and other receptors or markers on the tumor cell surface. Scientists discover new markers regularly. Which of these should be measured changes over time, based on current scientific research. The medical community is always seeking better ways to predict which patients are at risk for a recurrence of tumors so the patients who need further treatment can get it as soon as possible.

In summary, many factors must be weighed in deciding the treatment you'll receive. This is a crucial time to quiz your surgeon, discuss options with your family, and seek God. The choices are complex, but your doctor, your loved ones, and your God will help to see you through until you reach your destination.

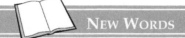 NEW WORDS

Bone scan: An imaging study that uses radioactive particles designed to show any areas where cancer cells are lodged in bones.

Capsular contracture: Scar tissue that develops around an implant, causing the breast to harden.

Collagen vascular disease: A group of illnesses associated with certain kinds of arthritis and other conditions.

Estrogen and progesterone receptors: Substances in cells that respond to the presence of estrogen or progesterone. In tumor cells, these receptors allow the cells to grow better if estrogen is present. Blocking these receptors when present can inhibit tumor growth. When tumor cells do not have these receptors, blocking estrogen has no effect on tumor growth.

     PART 2: THE MEDICAL JOURNEY

In situ: Cancer that has not yet invaded surrounding tissues.

Infiltrating lobular carcinoma: A type of breast cancer that has a tendency to be more diffuse (spread out) and subtle in the breast tissue compared to invasive duct carcinoma.

Invasive, or infiltrating, duct cancer: The most common type of breast cancer, originates in the duct system in the breast.

Liver sonogram: An imaging study of the liver using sound waves (ultrasonography).

Lobular carcinoma in situ: A premalignant condition that is associated with a higher than average incidence of breast cancer in either breast.

Markers: Compounds or substances, besides estrogen and progesterone receptors, on the surface of cancer cells or within the cells that can be measured to determine how aggressively a particular tumor might behave.

Metastatic disease: Cancer cells that have migrated and started to grow outside the site of the original tumor.

Multifocal disease: Cancer cells in multiple places within the breast.

Prophylactic mastectomy: Removal of the breast with no cancer present, done to prevent a subsequent breast cancer.

WHAT LOVED ONES CAN DO

As the patient prepares for surgery, her loved ones need to prepare as well. Each person responds to the stresses of this time in different ways; give each other room to be unique in your responses.

For example, some men prefer to wait alone during surgery. It affords them freedom not to have to be strong in the face of a difficult situation. Other men greatly appreciate the support of friends being with them. There is no right or wrong. Just be aware and tailor your actions to suit the close family.

Be available and supportive without being pushy. Once a patient makes a decision about treatment, refrain from giving advice, but be supportive. Questions such as, "Are you sure you're doing the right thing?" "Did you get a second opinion?" And "Why did you choose *that* surgery?" could cause insecurity in the patient at a time she needs to feel supported. If she asks your opinion, make sure she really wants it. Be careful how you phrase your thoughts. Realize that only the patient can make this decision that affects her and her future so profoundly.

Don't bombard the patient with questions about the prognosis. Details such as the size of the tumor, extent of cancer in the breast, and the status of the lymph nodes will come a few days after surgery.

Have someone help with visitors if needed (control unwanted visitors). Think ahead and designate this to an individual. The spouse or primary caretaker for the patient may have other obligations to attend to; this would be a job for a close friend or family member.

If the patient is recovering from surgery or any other treatment, a friend might help most by saying little or nothing. Most of the time the patient is expending her energy recovering and doesn't need pressure to entertain. Nor does the patient want to be entertained. (This varies according to the patient's personality.)

Do something fun on the way home from the hospital if mood and energy allow.

The best time to call or stop by to see a patient recovering from surgery may be a few days to a week or two after the surgery. Typically, people come by while the patient is in the hospital, but the days at home after the hospital stay can get lonely.

Don't ask the patient what you can do to help or ask her to call if she needs something. Rather, put yourself in her place and think of what you would like, then make a specific suggestion such as, "May I come clean your house tomorrow?" or "What time could I bring by dinner tonight?"

Tonya appreciated that her friends helped to bring some normalcy to her life by asking her to social events. "When our friends had a get-together, they would invite us, knowing I didn't feel well for long periods at a time. They might have a football party that lasted all afternoon. So they would make sure I could come, even if I only wanted to stay for an hour or so."

STRENGTHENING THOUGHTS FROM GOD'S WORD

"You have made known to me the path of life; you will fill me with joy in your presence, with eternal pleasures at your right hand" (Ps. 16:11).

"May your unfailing love rest upon us, O Lord, even as we put our hope in you" (Ps. 33:22).

"Show me the way I should go, for to you I lift up my soul" (Ps. 143:8).

CHAPTER 7

THE NEXT STEP: POST-SURGERY CHEMOTHERAPY AND HORMONE BLOCKER THERAPY

Once you've faced surgery, wouldn't it be great if your breast cancer journey were over? Unfortunately, surgery and radiation therapy treat only the cancer in the breast. But the entire body usually needs treatment because the cancer cells can escape from the breast and be too small to detect with any test.

At this point, your doctor may use the term "adjuvant therapy," which means treatment given as an adjunct, or in addition to, your surgery. Another phrase that might be used is "systemic therapy." This additional treatment could take the form of chemotherapy (usually administered as drugs in a vein) or hormonal blocker therapy (administered as oral medications) or both. The good news is that studies show an increased cure rate if these are done, even when no lymph nodes are involved with a tumor.[1]

While your mind understands the rationale for taking the treatment, I know that most patients view this phase with particular fear, especially regarding chemotherapy. In this chapter, we'll take a closer look at just what chemotherapy and hormone blocker therapy are and how they work. As in previous chapters, we'll hear from women who have experienced the treatments—what it was like for the women and how they felt about it.

THE MEDICAL ONCOLOGIST

After you've completed a lumpectomy or a mastectomy, the next step often is to see a medical oncologist who specializes in systemic therapy. He or she is part of your cancer team, along with the surgeon and radiation oncologist.

The first visit to the medical oncologist may well be your most anxiety-ridden experience. The oncologist generally goes over staging and cancer statistics with you. Realize that statistics pertain to what happened to others and are ballpark figures at best, not a glance into a crystal ball. The oncologist will also discuss side effects. The prospect of hair loss, nausea, and other side effects associated with chemotherapy can be daunting. Fortunately, patients tolerate chemotherapy better today because of new drugs that help to deal with these effects. As with surgery, the best place to get information is from your doctor rather than from friends or family, who have good intentions but often inaccurate information. Plus it's important to keep in mind that one person's experience can be radically different from another's, and just because a friend had a certain response to a treatment, it doesn't mean you will.

What Is Chemotherapy?

Chemotherapy drugs attack cells that divide rapidly. Often doctors recommend a combination of several drugs because the different drugs simultaneously attack the cells in different ways.

For chemotherapy to be effective, the dose and frequency given are very important. This became apparent in the 1980s, when an Italian research group reported that only patients who had received at least 85 percent of the intended chemotherapy dose showed a significant benefit, whereas patients receiving less than 65 percent had the same survival rate as those not receiving any chemotherapy.[2]

The specific drugs used, their timing, and the number of treatments is called a "protocol," "treatment regimen," or "treatment plan." Since researchers regularly discover and test new drugs, this book will not discuss any one protocol. Your medical oncologist will do that with you.

Typically, chemotherapy drugs are given over a few hours for a day or two and repeated every three weeks. These are called "cycles" or "courses" of chemotherapy. The first one usually is given within four to six weeks after the original surgery. Sometimes it's delayed, but it's preferable to start the cycle within eight weeks. The medical oncologist determines the number of cycles, which drugs are used, and the prescribed dosage. If the patient can't tolerate the side effects, the doctor will sometimes delay the cycle or reduce the dosage of a drug. Medications can be prescribed to reduce the side effects.

As Tonya faced chemotherapy, she needed help caring for her week-old baby. Her mother stepped in to help for seven months and, to make it easier for everyone, Tonya and the baby moved into her parents' home.

"Our faith at that time was the catalyst in the outcome of Tonya's horrific situation," said her mother, Nancy. "It was overwhelming to learn that your child has cancer at such a tender age with a new marriage, a baby on the way, and a career. As a grandparent as well as a parent, I wanted to be excited about the birth of our first grand-child, but we were wracked with fear for Tonya's health and what effect the cancer would have on the child. It was hard to stay focused and remain joyful at that time."

Tonya handled chemotherapy well. But after delivering her baby, she did have to deal with pneumonia and a blood clot in her lung that delayed her treatment a few weeks. Her oncologist suggested she would be a good candidate for a high-risk study, which she agreed to participate in. In this study only four chemotherapy treatments are given. They consist of three drugs, given in combination, that are 90 percent stronger than standard doses.

Chemotherapy came to be used as a cancer treatment back in the 1950s, when researchers observed that laboratory animals with a few tumor cells could at times be cured with chemotherapy, whereas delaying treatment could lead to an incurable situation. The first chemotherapy trial on breast cancer patients started in 1958.[3] These women had no known tumor cells outside the breast. In the 1960s and 1970s, most of the studies involved chemotherapy for one or two years, often with only a single drug. In the 1980s, more effective drugs were found, multiple drugs were used together, and chemotherapy began to be used in women without cancer cells in their lymph nodes. In the past decade, research has centered on how many courses of chemotherapy are necessary, whether higher doses are helpful, and whether chemotherapy given before surgery has any advantages over that given after surgery.

I WAS WONDERING . . .

During consultation with your medical oncologist, you should have covered the expected treatment, schedule, and drugs to be used, along with their side effects. Here are the questions that should have been answered:

- How long will each treatment last?
- Should I eat before I come?
- Should I expect to drive home or bring a driver with me?
- Can I take vitamins or herbs while on treatment?
- Can I utilize alternative medications or treatments?

JUST HOW BAD ARE THE SIDE EFFECTS?

Because normal cells as well as cancer cells divide, the chemotherapy drugs will affect both types. Fortunately, normal cells have a much greater ability to recover from the chemotherapy than do the malignant cells. Hair loss is common. The blood cells, the lining of the stomach, and the intestinal tract also are affected for the same reason. These side effects would diminish if the tumor cells themselves could be targeted without harming normal cells; so this has been an area of active research for many years.

"While I never actually got sick," Jane said, "I felt as if a huge lump was in my stomach. It just sat there for about a week after each chemo treatment.

"At my second chemo treatment, it took five pokes and three different technicians before they could get the IV line in. What a pain! I hadn't lost any hair yet. You wear an icecap to keep the drugs from getting into the cells at the base of the hair in hopes that this will keep it from breaking off. But when I took off the icecap, clumps of hair came out. What a depressing day!

"Eventually I did lose almost all my hair. I think that was the hardest for me because it was so visible.

"On the plus side, I didn't have to shave my legs for a while. I did wear a wig some, and it helped me to just forget the situation and not have people treat me differently. Our daughter was in high school and our son in junior high, and it was easier on them not to have to explain to their friends why Mom was wearing a bandana—a 'do rag' to them. I think the wigs today look pretty natural. As a matter of fact, I went to the hospital to visit one of our elderly church members (85 plus). I thought she had heard about my cancer and treatments, but when I walked in, Mrs. G said, 'I just love your hair shorter. I never did like long hair.' What was I going to say? I just said thanks."

Speaking of wigs, you're likely to want one, even if you wear it only on "special occasions." They are available at local hair salons, or you can find out who sells them by checking your yellow pages. If you can't afford a wig (some insurance companies will help to pay for them), check with a local cancer organization. Many survivors donate their wigs to such organizations.

Josefa used her hair loss to have some fun with her hairdresser. She normally visited the beauty shop almost every week. After her second treatment of chemotherapy, her hair was falling out. That Saturday, she went to her hair appointment as usual. When her stylist began to work, her hands became covered with Josefa's hair. Josefa pretended not to notice.

Her hairdresser finally asked, "What's happening? Each time I touch your head more hair comes out."

Josefa replied, "I don't know why this is happening. What kind of product did you use today as a conditioner?"

The flustered hairdresser quickly responded that she used the same conditioner as always.

"So you're sure it's not your fault?" Josefa questioned. Then, not able to contain herself any longer, she laughed and explained, "Many times when people are on chemo treatments, they lose their hair." Both had a good laugh.

Some of the other side effects are fragile mucous membranes resulting in mouth sores, changes in taste and smell, intestinal changes, headaches, dry skin, fatigue, memory loss, lowered concentration, and an increased risk of infections because your white cell blood count is lowered. These infections can be very serious, so precautions must be taken not to let the blood counts get too low and to try to stay away from individuals with contagious illnesses. But much of the risk of infection comes from within the patient, such as dental problems, sores in the mouth or elsewhere, or bladder infections.

Since white blood cells circulate in the blood and are produced in the bone marrow, in the 1990s drugs became available that stimulate the bone marrow to produce more white blood cells. When a patient takes these drugs in addition to the chemotherapy, she can receive higher doses without causing the white cells to get too low.[4] These drugs have helped to decrease hospital admissions for fever or infection. Also available are drugs to help increase the red blood cell count to diminish anemia.

Menopausal symptoms such as hot flashes are common during chemotherapy. The drugs used typically suppress ovarian production of estrogen and progesterone, and that production might not return after treatment in women still having periods at the time chemotherapy is started.

Because new drug combinations and timing sequences are always being researched, your doctor might ask you to participate in a clinical trial or research protocol. Clinical trials improve cancer care, and if you are eligible for one, your doctor or nurse will give you detailed written information about the study, risks and benefits to you, and what it will require of you.

WHY DO SOME WOMEN HAVE PORTS INSERTED?

Most chemotherapy drugs are given in the vein, so some oncologists recommend that you have an indwelling catheter (also called a "port") inserted. This requires a surgical procedure in which a small tube is placed in a large vein near the neck and attached to an injection site, which is put under the skin below the collarbone. When chemotherapy is given, the skin over the port is anesthetized and the needle is placed into the port. This procedure prevents a patient from having a catheter inserted into a vein in the arm each time. The need for a port varies based on the patient's circumstances, the number of cycles, and the oncologist's methods.

Jody received a port and described her first chemotherapy this way: "Today we went in to the chemo office around 8:30 A.M. They drew blood from the port, and let me tell you, it was the easiest blood I have ever had drawn. Then we watched two videos about chemotherapy and had personalized education from one of the chemo nurses. All this was done while we waited for my blood work to be analyzed so they could personalize the chemo to fit my body. (Imagine that! I have custom-made chemicals.) After the lab results were back, they started the IVs. They took a long time. I'm supposed to drink lots of liquids—three quarts a day—at least for the first three days after treatment."

What Is a Normal Response to the Treatments?

Most women continue to work during chemotherapy and may even find it helps them to maintain as normal a schedule as possible. You can expect some fatigue while on the treatment. That might mean a lightened schedule or reduced work hours. Often you need to go through a couple of cycles to see what level of activity is realistic for you. But studies show that exercise increases energy levels.

Because you don't know what to expect with chemotherapy, particularly the first couple of times it's given, you may put up with symptoms that your doctor can control with medications. No two women are alike or respond to chemotherapy the same. Don't hesitate to call your medical oncologist or oncology nurse if something unexpected occurs after treatment. They may be able to help you feel much better.

Jody experienced severe nausea, headaches, and insomnia after her first chemotherapy. "I couldn't remember ever being so sick," she said. Her doctor found the blend of drugs was creating these side effects and made adjustments before the second treatment. After the second treatment, Jody felt knocked out by the medications and couldn't stay awake for any length of time, but the sleep wasn't restful and seemed unnatural. Once again the balance of drugs was changed. "I'm happy to report that I had a much better reaction," Jody said of the third treatment. "I wasn't as 'out of it,' and even though I slept a lot, it was a natural sleep. When I was awake, I was tired but only had a little queasiness."

Jody's experience points out how important it is to communicate the side effects you're having. At first Jody didn't tell her doctor how sick she was because she felt having "poisons" pumped into her system would result in feeling bad, so why tell anyone? As a result, her doctor wasn't able to work with her as quickly as possible to help her to deal with the symptoms. And when she was so sick, it was hard for her to communicate all her symptoms.

PRACTICAL SUGGESTIONS

While undergoing chemotherapy, don't make significant weight changes. If you were beginning a diet, postpone it until the treatment is finished. You may even gain weight with chemotherapy because of the reduced activity level, hormonal changes, and the tendency to eat to settle your stomach.

If you're feeling anxious the evening prior to chemotherapy, plan something fun that evening. Go to a movie, eat out, visit friends, or do something else you enjoy.

One patient chose to have chemotherapy late in the day but early in the week so that by the weekend she could feel well enough to do fun things with friends. Having that goal to look forward to helped her through the week. While you might not be up to doing everything as before, within the limits of energy available, go for it!

Friends sometimes try to discourage your getting together with others, thinking they are doing you a favor and protecting you from exposure to illness. While that is true for a few days each treatment cycle when you are particularly vulnerable to infection, most of the time this is not the case. If you are not sure about when those vulnerable times are occurring, ask your oncology nurse or doctor.

Try to complete dental work prior to starting chemotherapy. Cavities can lead to infections that could fester during chemotherapy.

Ask family or friends to take you to your first chemotherapy and stay with you at least the first day. After the first time, you'll have a better feel about what to expect.

Believing in the usefulness of chemotherapy will help get you through it.

Find creative ways to bring humor and enjoyable activities into your daily life. Perhaps you could ask friends to send cards, cartoons they especially enjoyed, or to find other lighthearted ways to support you.

"The most traumatic thing about chemo was the first treatment," Sandy recounted. "Nothing scared me as much. I was so terrified I couldn't pray. I did a deep breathing exercise, and I was trying not to cry. After the first chemo, I wasn't afraid anymore. I knew the drill; it was just one more notch in my gun of courage."

AREAS OF CHEMOTHERAPY RESEARCH

Bone marrow transplants are being researched in which a patient has bone marrow tissue removed or stem cells drawn from a large vein. This tissue is stored. Then the patient is given very high doses of chemotherapy, enough to kill all the white cells. The hope is that the high blood levels of drugs, maintained for a short time, will kill tumor cells resistant to lower drug doses. A few days after the drugs are given, the patient receives back the bone marrow or stem cells, and recovery begins. This procedure requires several weeks in the hospital and has many side effects. In 1998, several studies failed to demonstrate that the treatment was beneficial to breast cancer patients.[5] Researchers continue to explore whether a select group of patients might benefit.

Researchers also are studying a growth factor receptor called Her2/neu, which is found in approximately 20 percent of breast cancers. The receptors on a cell's outside surface provide a way to potentially distinguish between cancerous and normal cells. If the receptors are present in abnormally high numbers on the surface of cancer cells, they may act as part of a signaling system that tells the cancer cells to divide. An antibody called Herceptin was developed to block these receptors. Early studies showed that in about 20 percent of the patients receiving Herceptin, tumors diminished.[6] Combining certain chemotherapy drugs with Herceptin increases the cancer-killing power of the drugs. But Herceptin may also cause heart problems in a few patients. So research continues on when and how to use this drug.

It might seem like a simple task to determine whether treatment with a particular drug is useful in preventing a recurrence of breast cancer. Why not treat several new patients and see whether they do better than previous patients (called "historic controls")?

But breast cancer behaves differently in different patients. Sometimes it grows very fast; at other times the tumor grows more slowly and is less aggressive. Although we know these tumors all start from the breast tissue, some tumor cells have estrogen receptors and others do not. Some tumor cells have a greater ability to migrate into the lymph or blood vessels and thus spread outside the breast. Tumor cells also differ in their response to chemotherapy from one person to the next and even within the same tumor. Breast cancer cells seem to be as unique as the individuals in which they develop. Because of these varying biological characteristics, breast cancer treatment must be individualized. This also means that clear answers about the effectiveness of differing treatments are tricky to obtain.

Studies have been designed to take into account these differences and compensate for them. The most accurate way to do this is a randomized trial. This means that once a patient meets certain criteria, she is assigned randomly to one of two or more treatment groups. Neither the doctor nor the patient chooses which group to enter. When many patients participate in the study, most of the factors that could cause false impressions are minimized. For instance, you would expect that the two groups would have about the same number of highly aggressive tumors, and the age range would be about the same. This allows for a fairer comparison of the two treatment options.

New drug development is a hot area of research. Researchers develop new chemotherapy drugs in three phases. If your doctor asks you to participate in a research protocol, it is almost certainly a phase-three study, which means that the drug has proven its effectiveness, and dosing with tolerable side effects has already been established.

In the phase-three trial, researchers compare the new drug or treatment protocol to the prevailing standard treatment. The new treatment is believed to be at least as effective as the standard treatment, perhaps more effective. Just the dosing, timing, and combinations of drugs are being adjusted. The study may be blinded, meaning that you and your doctor will not know which treatment you are on. Studies done in this fashion are essential to an accurate and unbiased understanding of which treatments are best for cancer patients.

The more patients who are willing to participate, the faster answers will come. Currently, only about 4 percent of breast cancer patients are enrolled in randomized clinical trials.[7] At every hospital offering such research studies, a committee makes sure any study is safe and reasonable, and that the patient is fully informed.

In addition to being aware of research that you might participate in, you need to understand the difference between absolute and relative differences in results. Knowing the difference will help you to sort out health information reported in the news media or discussed with your medical team.

Let's suppose that without any treatment, patients have a 90 percent chance of no tumor recurrence. That means ten out of one hundred patients will have recurrence and ninety will not. In a second group that employed a particular treatment, a 95 percent chance of no recurrence was found. That means ninety patients wouldn't have had a recurrence anyway and five recurrences were prevented. This would be reported as a 50 percent relative improvement in cure rate. That's because in the first group, ten patients had recurrences; in the second group five had recurrences. Five recurrences were prevented, which is 50 percent of the ten expected recurrences. The *absolute* difference is 5 percent. That is, five people out of a hundred taking the treatment had a recurrence prevented.

When new medical treatments are discussed in the news media, often the *relative* difference is the only number given. It sounds much more dramatic to report a 50 percent difference than a 5 percent difference. So the results from a new treatment might seem more significant than they really are. When you read of potential new treatments, ask your doctor whether the test results indicate something that might be a good treatment for you.

HORMONAL THERAPY

What function does hormonal therapy have in treating breast cancer? Normal breast tissue cells have receptors for both progesterone and estrogen. They cause normal breast tissue to grow and mature properly. But when a cell becomes cancerous, it may retain some of the characteristics of a normal breast tissue cell, such as the receptors, or it may lose them. If cancer cells have these receptors, blocking them may inhibit tumor growth. That's one reason tumors are tested for the presence of these receptors.

Most women past menopause will have these receptors in their tumor cells. Younger women are less likely to have the receptors.

Most of the hormone-blocking medications are oral drugs that "block" the effects of estrogen on the tumor cells. If the tumor cells have the estrogen receptors, blocking those receptors with drugs can be a very effective way of suppressing the tumor.

The drug Tamoxifen, the most widely studied drug of this type, has been in use for more than thirty years. You would probably take it for five years. In addition to suppressing breast cancer, it also helps to maintain bone density and may have a beneficial effect on blood cholesterol levels. Side effects include menopausal symptoms such as hot flashes, mood swings, decreased libido, and vaginal dryness. Because it stimulates the uterine lining, women who have not had a hysterectomy have a small risk of developing uterine cancer. For that reason, it's important to see your gynecologist at least annually and to report any vaginal bleeding quickly.

Jane, who took Tamoxifen, experienced hot flashes, which she described as "making me want to jump out of my skin—or at least my clothes." When she had a hot flash, she couldn't concentrate. And the flare-ups would wake her at night, making it difficult to get a good night's sleep.

Most hormonal medications, such as birth control pills, hormone replacement therapy, and antiestrogens such as Tamoxifen, are all associated with a small risk of deep vein clots. If these form in large veins in the pelvis, they can travel to the lung and cause serious problems. The risk seems to be about the same regardless of which type of hormonal medication a woman takes. Women who previously took estrogen for years without developing deep vein clots should be no more likely to have clots with Tamoxifen than with the previous estrogen.

Most researchers believe the benefit of taking Tamoxifen outweighs the risks. Vigorous research is under way to find similar drugs that have fewer side effects. A number of selective estrogen receptor modulators (SERMs) are in the research lab and now are entering clinical trials. Another class of drugs, called aromatase inhibitors, is also in studies. These drugs, which work to stop estrogen production, have resulted in favorable preliminary reports, with effectiveness similar to Tamoxifen, but are less likely to cause blood clots.

So there you have it. At this point both chemotherapy and hormone-blocking medications provide long-term, positive results that are well worth the temporary discomfort they can cause. Just ask the women who have made it through this part of the journey. Jody was in a celebratory mood when she had her port removed; she felt freed from the last vestige that reminded her of chemo. She had "graduated," and you will, too.

In the next chapter, we'll look at radiation therapy and explore who receives it, what the experience is like, and what the side effects are.

What Loved Ones Can Do

For friends, remember that if the patient is nauseated, bringing in food for the rest of the family may be more appreciated now than during surgery. It helps the patient stay out of the kitchen.

Sometimes simple acts speak loudly. Jane recalls something simple her husband did that really touched her. "The day after the chemo treatment, I realized it was time to plant pansies in our front yard. In Texas they'll last all winter if you get them in at the right time to root well. But I couldn't put them out due to the fatigue and low immune system. My sweet husband, who really doesn't like gardening, planted them for me. It really helped at that point to bring a little normalcy to an abnormal situation. And knowing that he cared was even more important in lifting my spirits."

Saying the right words of encouragement during a patient's vulnerable moment can make an immense difference. Tonya related the following story: "I remember taking a shower, and my hair had really gotten dead. It had not actually broken off or come out completely. But I remember standing in the bathroom, with my hair falling out, and I was in tears. I looked at my husband and said, 'Look at me! I have one boob, and I'm bald, and I'm just ugly!' He put his arms around me and said, 'Baby, you're still as beautiful as you ever were.' I didn't believe him, but we both started to giggle, and suddenly I felt better and very loved."

Karen dealt with her hair loss by asking a friend to come over and shave Karen's head. "I decided to be proactive. Rather than let my hair fall out, I just shaved it off. I went out and bought hats or scarves in every color to go with all my outfits. A bunch of my friends and I got together, and we used a digital camera to record a fashion show with all my outfits."

 New Words

Absolute differences: The actual number of patients benefiting from a treatment.

Adjuvant therapy: Chemotherapy or hormonal therapy used after surgery to diminish chances of cancer recurrence.

Blinded study: The patient and sometimes the physician don't know what treatment the patient is taking so that evaluation of benefit and side effects will not be influenced by that knowledge.

Chemotherapy course: One episode of treatment with chemotherapy drugs, usually a combination of several drugs.

Chemotherapy protocol: A plan describing the timing and types of drugs to be used for a particular patient receiving chemotherapy.

Cycles of chemotherapy: Same as a course of chemotherapy.

Historic controls: Patients who didn't receive the treatment being studied.

Randomized trial: A study in which patients are randomly assigned to a treatment group in an attempt to assure that the groups are similar in every respect except the different treatments.

Relative differences: The percentage difference of patients benefiting from a treatment.

Systemic therapy: Treatment to the entire body, typically referring to chemotherapy or hormonal therapy.

STRENGTHENING THOUGHTS
FROM GOD'S WORD

"Your Father knows what you need before you ask him" (Matt. 6:8).

"Let us then approach the throne of grace with confidence, so that we may receive mercy and find grace to help us in our time of need" (Heb. 4:16).

CHAPTER 8

MOVING ONWARD: RADIATION THERAPY

Most people are familiar with radiation and are aware it pervades our environment. But the thought of being radiated disturbs most patients. Do you become a menace to yourself and your family? How is the radiation administered? Why is it necessary? What are the side effects? Are long-term effects something to worry about? These are the questions we'll take a look at in this chapter.

Therapeutic radiation consists of an invisible, high-energy wave-particle structure similar to the radiation used for diagnostic films, such as a mammogram, but at a much greater intensity. Radiation treatments can be localized to a particular area where cancer cells are found and are considered a type of local therapy, like surgery. You'll be relieved to know that it usually doesn't cause nausea, hair loss, or other symptoms people associate with cancer therapy.

Why Do I Need Radiation Therapy?

Radiation therapy damages the cancer cell's DNA so the cell can't repair itself. If a cell can't be repaired within twenty-four hours, it dies. Radiation targets cells that are dividing, such as malignant cells. Normal cells that might be damaged by the radiation have a greater ability to make repairs than cancer cells. As a result, radiation "kills" cancer cells while normal cells rejuvenate.

What Is the Treatment Like?

Typically you will lie down in a specific position for about ten minutes to receive the daily treatment. Most of those ten minutes are spent in precise positioning so each treatment will accurately target the area to be radiated and to make sure the same area is radiated each time. The actual radiation takes only a few moments and usually is administered at the same time each day. You receive the treatment every weekday for six or seven weeks. Radiation starts three or four weeks after you've completed chemotherapy or surgery (if no chemotherapy is needed). The radiation therapist is the person you'll see every day who positions you and tends to any of your needs.

How Much Radiation Is Used?

When treating cancer, doctors use radiation in doses more than a thousand times higher than that employed for diagnostic films. This dose causes cells that are dividing in the area radiated to die. The same dose is delivered each day.

What Steps Do I Go Through as the Treatment Begins?

A specially trained and board-certified physician, called a radiation oncologist, plans and oversees the radiation therapy. Before the treatments start, you'll consult with this physician to determine if you need radiation and to give you a chance to ask any questions you might have. For this appointment, be sure to take a complete set of records, including pathology reports, any X-rays, and a complete medical history with a list of medications. This will be a time you'll be glad that you kept your medical notebook because all this information will be readily available. If you've had any radiation previously, the radiation oncologist will need those medical records. You can obtain them from the place where the initial radiation was given.

Some of the questions you'll want to ask include:

- What do you expect the radiation to do to my cancer?
- Will I need treatment beyond radiation? If so, what will that be?
- How will I feel while I'm receiving the treatment?
- Will this affect my ability to work?
- What are the side effects and how long will they last?
- What is likely to happen if I choose not to have radiation?
- How will the area being radiated be marked?

A few days prior to starting the radiation therapy, you'll have a second appointment with the radiation oncologist for a treatment simulation. Your position during the treatments will be arranged, and X-rays will be taken in the treatment position to help the radiation oncologist plan the best way to deliver the radiation. The machine used during the simulation looks like the radiation equipment, but it's only for planning purposes. Several films or a CT scan are taken and calculations are made so that the precise area requiring radiation is accurately targeted.

WHY DO I HAVE TO HAVE SKIN MARKS?

The area radiated will be exactly the same each day. That's why careful planning is done. Marks are placed on the skin for the same reason. Sometimes the marks are permanent tattoos, and sometimes temporary marks are used and carefully maintained from day to day. The radiation therapist must be able to align the breast accurately every day for the radiation to be successful. Whether permanent or temporary marks are used is a point of discussion between you and your radiation oncologist.

The marks are dots, and while you might find it shocking that you could be tattooed, keep in mind that positioning of the radiation is critical. And, yes, the tattoos can be removed after the treatments are over. But should you ever need radiation again, the positioning of this series of radiation treatments is critical to know. Once women understand this, they often decide to view the tattoos as a lifetime safeguard.

After this simulation appointment, the radiation oncologist will see you weekly during therapy or at any time a question or problem arises that needs the physician's input.

WHAT DOES RADIATION FEEL LIKE?

During radiation therapy, the breast or chest wall often becomes swollen, tender, and red. The skin may be itchy, look sunburned, and may peel. The equipment used for radiation can also make a difference in the dosage delivered to the skin. Once again, everyone is different in what the experience is like for her.

Karen, who is fair-skinned, experienced fairly severe burns during the treatment. Toward the end of radiation, she felt pretty uncomfortable because of the burns and couldn't wear a bra. But she never missed a day of work.

Lola described radiation as "a breeze." She had minor burns because she, too, is fair-skinned. But she wasn't tired and realized she was near the end of her treatments—and that brightened her up considerably.

Jody was emotionally unprepared for the experience. She thought the treatment would consist of a single zap, but she had four blasts each time. "My skin did well," she reported, "and I didn't have any real problem with rashes, but I did have a few burns by the end." What really caught her off guard was that she felt tired from the beginning of the treatment. "I thought the hard part was over, having made it through surgery and chemo, and now I could get back to 'normal.'" Dealing with the disappointment of not having much energy was the biggest challenge for her.

Ask your radiation doctor for help if you have skin problems during radiation. Some home remedies might not work or might even worsen the problem.

Like Jody, you could feel fatigue while on the radiation, but this usually isn't severe enough to alter your daily activities. The fatigue will slowly increase during radiation and may persist several weeks to months after the treatments are over.

Although rare, some women notice a dry cough three to five weeks after the treatments are finished due to the radiation affecting lung tissue just behind the breast. This may persist for several weeks but usually clears up without specific treatment. About one in 200 women might experience this. One in ten women receiving chemotherapy at the same time as the radiation develop the cough.

Also keep in mind that stress may come from the change in your schedule that radiation could require, or from fear, or from any number of individual challenges. These things can lead to depression. Recognizing the source of these emotions can help you to cope. This is normal and best handled one day at a time. Facing the irritations and issues as they come is better than bottling them up, when they might pop out unexpectedly. We'll discuss the emotional side of your breast cancer journey more in chapter 10.

Will Radiation Make Me Radioactive?

Radiation therapy will not make you radioactive or pose any danger to others you come in contact with. It does cause permanent changes in the tissues radiated. Increased pigmentation in the skin may be permanent. You should protect the treated skin from sun exposure for up to eighteen months after radiation. Rib fractures occur after chest wall radiation in about one in 250 women—even years later.

Are There Any Long-Term Effects of the Radiation?

The breast might swell during therapy or could gradually reduce in size with time due to scarring, or "fibrosis," a general hardening of the tissue. Months or years after the radiation is complete, the breast may be firmer as a result of fibrosis.

After radiation therapy, the blood supply to the area isn't as resilient as before. Because of the permanent change in the area, radiation therapy usually is done only once. The changes rarely cause a problem, but can affect subsequent surgery to that breast. If a woman decides to have a mastectomy and breast reconstruction years after her lumpectomy, this can be more difficult because of the decreased blood supply.

Malignancies can arise within areas of previous radiation, but this is rare (from one woman in 500 to one in 3,000). Most of these are sarcomas, a different kind of malignancy than breast cancer, which can occur five to twenty years later.

Can Radiation Therapy Prevent Breast Cancer?

If radiation therapy kills cancer cells, can it prevent breast cancer? Premalignant changes in the breast, such as atypical duct hyperplasia or lobular carcinoma in situ (LCIS), may be found through a breast biopsy. Both of these changes in the breast tissue suggest a higher risk of developing breast cancer, but don't require immediate treatment. Would radiation therapy decrease the likelihood of breast cancer in these situations? Unfortunately, no scientific evidence shows that to be the case.

IF I HAD A LUMPECTOMY, WILL I NEED RADIATION?

When you have a lumpectomy, even if the edges, or margins, of the tumor area are free of cancer cells, studies show 40 percent of women have recurrences.[1] That's because microscopic tumor cells were still in the remaining breast tissue but were undetectable. Therapeutic radiation kills tumor cells that may remain in the breast or surrounding tissues following a lumpectomy and therefore is often used after a lumpectomy.

Surgeons used lumpectomy for hundreds of years without successfully eradicating breast cancer. Discovering radiation and refining the use of it has made lumpectomy an option for breast cancer treatment. With a lumpectomy, only a small dose of radiation is given each day, and the treatment continues for several weeks.

IS RADIATION EVER USED AS THE ONLY TREATMENT FOR CANCER?

If radiation can kill tumor cells, then why not use radiation alone, without surgery? The French were the first of many to explore that option in the 1950s,[2] but they found that much more radiation was necessary to kill tumors large enough to see or feel. Doses 20 to 30 percent higher were needed to kill large numbers of cancer cells as opposed to the microscopic cells that remain after a lumpectomy. With those high doses, large amounts of scar tissue and even ulceration occurred, sometimes years after the radiation.

Can I Wait to See If I Have a Recurrence after My Lumpectomy?

If 60 percent of women having a lumpectomy don't have recurrences when no radiation is given, why not wait until a tumor recurs? Because tumor cells could escape from the breast and lodge elsewhere in the body if you do have a recurrence. Also, by the time cancer can be found on a mammogram or through a breast exam, it already involves millions or billions of cells. More radiation therapy would be required resulting in a poorer cosmetic outcome. Waiting for a recurrence also lowers the chances of killing all the cancer cells. The best time to thoroughly and effectively treat cancer is when it's first discovered.

We now know that the combination of surgical removal of a tumor followed by radiation therapy yields the best cosmetic results, the fewest complications, and the best tumor control.

How Are the Radiated Areas Selected?

Sometimes the lymph node areas immediately surrounding the breast are radiated, and the lumpectomy site often receives slightly more radiation than the rest of the breast, but the entire breast is radiated. The higher dosage for the lumpectomy area is called a "boost." Since most recurrences are around the area where the tumor was removed, that area receives the slightly higher dosage. This has been very successful in destroying possible tumor cells and preventing a tumor from coming back in the breast. Even with radiation therapy, a tumor may recur in the breast in as many as 10 percent of women even ten years after treatment.

How Long Will I Have Radiation If I've Had a Lumpectomy?

Most lumpectomy patients will receive five weeks of radiation to the entire breast followed by a week or a week and a half of the boost at the site of the lumpectomy. The surgeon often marks the tumor area with small metallic clips at the time of the lumpectomy so that this area can be targeted accurately. These clips are imperceptible to you, and there is no need to remove them. They mark the area where the cancer was removed for future follow-up.

The boost is usually done with external radiation, similar to the first five weeks of treatment. But another technique involves radioactive implants placed through catheters (small tubes). These are placed surgically through the lumpectomy incision, and later loaded with the radioactive beads that stay in place for two or three days. An active area of research is the use of this latter technique for the entire radiation treatment. With this approach the catheters are inserted through one-third of the breast volume and stay in place for four or five days. To use this technique, you'll have to be hospitalized while the radioactive seeds are in place.

An alternative radiation technique called "high dose radiation" is also being investigated. In this technique the radiation is delivered to the local lumpectomy site through catheters or balloons inserted in the incision. Once the treatments are completed, the catheters or balloons are easily removed as an outpatient procedure.

If I Had a Mastectomy ...

Why would I need radiation therapy?

You might need radiation therapy for your chest wall even after a mastectomy. Radiation is recommended for large or diffuse (spread out) tumors, for a tumor close to the muscle behind the breast, or if several lymph nodes have cancer. Your physicians will discuss with you the particular reason radiation therapy is recommended for you.

When would I have radiation therapy?

After completing chemotherapy, most patients will move on to radiation therapy. Some institutions sandwich the radiation in the middle of chemotherapy. Chest wall radiation may also be done months or years after a mastectomy if the tumor comes back.

What side effects would I experience?

The skin often becomes quite red and sensitive during the weeks when the chest wall is treated. Tumor cells could be in or near the skin, so the radiation is designed to treat the skin as well as the underlying muscle and the lymph node areas around the chest.

Under what other conditions might I benefit from radiation therapy?

Breast cancer can spread through the bloodstream to other sites and sometimes is found outside the breast, as in bones around the spine or in the pelvis. When this occurs, radiation therapy may help to relieve pain or other symptoms. This radiation therapy often is two to three weeks in duration, again given daily. Your medical oncologist works closely with the radiation oncologist to determine when this is necessary.

Can radiation cause other cancers?

Can radiation cause other cancers outside the original irradiated field? Concern about the other breast, the one not being radiated, naturally arises. Fortunately, studies consistently show no increased risk of a second malignancy in the chest cavity or in the opposite breast or of leukemia after breast radiation.[3] However, women who smoke may have an increased risk of developing lung cancer after radiation therapy.

For many women who have radiation therapy, this is the last of the disruptive treatments they must receive for breast cancer. Once these are completed, you truly have reached your destination: a return to good health and your normal routines. It's time to celebrate! One woman took a trip to Hawaii with her husband to mark the occasion. Another woman was happy to return to life-before-breast-cancer, but did take the opportunity to gather friends around her to give thanks and party.

But reaching this point in your trip through breast cancer doesn't mean cancer has no residual effects. In the next chapters, we'll discuss how cancer touches your family, including your children, and your friends; how to restore your fitness and well-being; how alternative healing methods can fit into your regimen; and what you can do with the emotions that come attached to the pronouncement of breast cancer—and sometimes don't make themselves known until after the medical part of your journey is over.

WHAT LOVED ONES CAN DO

For some women, radiation therapy is more difficult than chemotherapy because of the daily routine required. If friends are available even occasionally to accompany the patient, it makes the time more pleasant. Do something fun afterwards, but even if there isn't time for that, the presence of a friend means a lot.

Buy bubble gum–flavored toothpaste for your friend; radiation causes a lack of saliva, and the gentle children's flavors of toothpaste are the most palatable.

Help your friend shop for a cotton-blend sports bra. Often radiation makes the breast very sensitive, and wearing a regular bra isn't always an option.

Supply your loved one with some musical tapes that you know she'll enjoy. She'll have to wait a long time for the equipment to be set up correctly, and listening to soothing music can help her to pass the time.

You might consider marking the completion of treatment with a celebration or surprise party. This is a big-time graduation for the breast cancer patient. A coronation for the "Queen with Mettle" might be a fun event.

New Words

Boost: Additional radiation to the lumpectomy site.

Catheters: Hollow tubes that allow insertion of radioactive material.

Fibrosis of the breast: Thickening and hardening of breast tissue.

Radioactive implants: Tiny radiation seeds placed through catheters directly within cancerous tissue or tumors to kill cancerous cells.

Strengthening Thoughts from God's Word

"I am still confident of this: I will see the goodness of the Lord in the land of the living. Wait for the Lord; be strong and take heart and wait for the Lord" (Ps. 27:13–14).

"We wait in hope for the Lord; he is our help and our shield. In him our hearts rejoice, for we trust in his holy name. May your unfailing love rest upon us, O Lord, even as we put our hope in you" (Ps. 33:20–22).

"My soul finds rest in God alone; my salvation comes from him" (Ps. 62:1).

CHAPTER 9

ALTERNATIVE HEALING METHODS

When you find you have a serious illness such as breast cancer, you wonder what options beyond conventional medical treatments are available to you. Do alternative healing methods offer beneficial options either complementary to traditional treatments or separate from them?

Humans are complex creations, and medical science is a rapidly advancing body of knowledge. As new discoveries are made, the appreciation of that complexity grows. What were thought to be simple systems are found to be far more complex than initially discerned. Some of what is now considered complementary or alternative medicine may well be incorporated into conventional medicine in years to come as more research sheds light on these treatments or methods.

At this point, what is clear is that not only are human beings marvelously created but the environment around them also is complex and sophisticated. Plants make all sorts of chemicals that can be useful or harmful. The relationships that exist between creatures and the environment make a fascinating study. The relationships of compounds within foods may be as important as the individual components of that food. Isolating vitamins or other compounds from the foods they are found in might not be as effective as a group of compounds normally found in food. Understanding plants and other components of the environment is still in its infancy.

We do know that stress reduction promotes recovery. Find what alleviates stress for you. Some women enjoy soaking in the bathtub, surrounded by bubbles, soft music, and candlelight. Bible reading, particularly the Psalms, can have a calming and relaxing effect as the mind is directed away from the immediate circumstances to God and his ways. Sipping a soothing tea in front of a fireplace and reading a book or a magazine help one to slip away from present concerns.

But what about the more "radical" approaches to dealing with breast cancer? Are certain foods or herbs able to stave off wildly increasing cancer cells?

A cancer survivor had this to say about the many options other people suggest to a person with cancer: "One of the most irritating things about getting cancer is that all of a sudden people start giving advice. It seems everyone has a theory on why you got it and how to cure it. Bookshelves are lined with the latest fad cures. Everywhere you look, the enlightened offer theories about why we gave ourselves cancer. Destructive and painful, this attitude helps friends convince themselves that they won't get cancer because they don't have our flaw—pick one of the latest (high fat, didn't exercise, stressed out, whatever). . . . Now, I am a strong proponent of complementary healing. These are things we do in addition to medicine—they aren't alternatives to medicine. I think cancer survivors have to take control, and that means finding ways to get healthy—stress reduction, nutrition, . . . vitamins. Hey, whatever works for you."

As a doctor, I would agree that the woman with breast cancer should take part in the healing process in whatever way makes sense to her—but she should always involve her doctor. The disease you're fighting is complex and mean. It's unlikely one "magic bullet" is going to take care of the problem, as much as we all wish that could be the case. Your doctor needs to know what vitamins, minerals, or herbs you're taking because many of them create a volatile "cocktail" when combined with prescribed medications.

Now let's take a look at some of the options purported to help you win the battle against breast cancer. (If you would like to explore these options in greater detail, you might read Dr. Walt Larimore and Donal O'Mathúna's *Alternative Medicine: The Christian Handbook.*[1])

BIOLOGICAL-BASED THERAPIES

Biological-based therapies may provide an adjunct to traditional cancer therapy. A few of the methods include:

ANTIOXIDANTS

These are chemical compounds found in many fruits and vegetables that might reduce cancer development by neutralizing free radicals. "Free radicals" are biologic chemicals found in tissues that are very active compounds and may cause damage to normal cells.

COENZYME Q_{10}

Also known as Co-Q_{10}, this is an antioxidant and coenzyme (helps enzymes to function properly). It is naturally produced by the body and promotes energy production in cells and prevention of oxidation of compounds on the cell surface. It has been studied since the 1960s and enjoyed considerable popularity for a number of years. Studies done in the 1960s showed decreased blood levels of the compound in cancer patients, stimulating further research to determine if it is useful in preventing or treating cancer. Although several studies did suggest it benefited cancer patients, problems with the design of the studies cast doubt on the results. It's considered possible, but not proven, that coenzyme Q_{10} inhibits tumor growth and prolongs survival from cancer.

Co-Q_{10} also might protect the heart from damage caused by cancer chemotherapy drugs since some drugs, such as Adriamycin, can affect the heart muscle. Animal studies showed a benefit with Co-Q_{10}, and several small studies on cancer patients have also suggested a benefit. Research is ongoing for this potential use. Co-Q_{10} is thought to be safe, but does interact with some other medications and compounds such as blood thinners. If you take this compound, be sure your treating physicians know.

CALCIUM D-GLUCARATE

Also called glucarate, this compound is found in fruits and vegetables. Animal studies showed some reduction in breast cancer tumors, but reliable studies in humans are lacking.

MELATONIN

A natural hormone produced by the body that has been connected with sleep cycles, melatonin also is an antioxidant.

SELENIUM

A mineral with antioxidant properties, it is found in whole grains and nuts and is an essential nutrient needed in small quantities in humans. Observations showed that geographic regions with a high soil content of selenium enjoyed a lower cancer mortality than regions with a low content. Research was done to determine if selenium had a role in cancer prevention or treatment. One study suggested that prostate, colon, and lung cancers occurred less frequently in the group taking selenium. Few women were included in that study, so no information about the incidence of breast cancer was produced. Other studies haven't been as encouraging, so more studies are needed before any conclusion can be drawn.

High intake of selenium can be toxic, resulting in hair and nail loss, skin lesions, weakness, and even kidney damage or harm to the immune system. Obviously, moderation is in order if you decide to supplement your treatment with this mineral.

SHARK CARTILAGE

Because sharks didn't seem to develop cancer, this part of their bodies has been studied over the past decade. But, in fact, sharks do develop cancer. Yet this belief resulted in studies that did yield some useful information. It appears that cartilage may slow down or prevent formation of new blood vessels in tissues. The formation of new blood vessels is essential for cancers to grow. Despite this fact, several studies, mostly with small numbers of patients, have failed to show a benefit for cancer patients who consumed shark cartilage. A compound isolated from shark cartilage currently is being tested in laboratories for anticancer activity. Since there are no adverse effects from taking shark cartilage, aside from those associated with consuming large quantities of a less-than-palatable substance, such as nausea, you could supplement your cancer treatment with this product.

MACROBIOTIC DIETS

These are strict vegetarian diets based on Chinese medical traditions. Typically whole grains and raw vegetables are consumed with beans, soybeans, nuts, and seeds. Fish may be consumed on occasion, but no meat or dairy products are allowed. This results in increasing fiber, reducing calories, and increasing wholesome vegetable intake, but dietary deficiencies can occur. Vitamin B_{12} is the most notable deficiency that could develop. No evidence of cancer cures or anticancer effect has been found in the macrobiotic diets.

SOY

Diets containing high soy intake have an unclear role in breast cancer. Asian countries where soy products have been used in high concentrations for generations have traditionally enjoyed a much lower incidence of breast cancer. But research regarding soy products hasn't been conclusive. High soy diets aren't recommended currently, and further research is ongoing.

HERBS

GREEN TEA

Made from the leaves of the *Camellia sinensis* plant, green tea comes in caffeinated and decaffeinated compounds. It has been purported to decrease the incidence of some cancers, including breast cancer. This isn't yet proven, but studies are under way to evaluate a possible benefit.

ESSIAC

This tea is composed of several plants, including burdock root, elm bark, rhubarb, and others. Several institutions have attempted to show it benefits cancer patients, but no consistently positive results have been reported.

OTHER TEAS AND HERBS

Some popular teas or herbs such as ginseng, Ginkgo biloba, ginger, and garlic are associated with increased bleeding tendencies and therefore aren't recommended prior to surgery. You would be wise to avoid these substances two weeks before your operation. But ginger root has a proven benefit for nausea and can even help with chemotherapy-induced nausea.

MILK THISTLE

This herb contains an antioxidant called silymarin that has been reported to help the liver—and perhaps to protect it—during chemotherapy. It has been used medicinally for two thousand years, and no serious adverse effects have been attributed to it. But no formal studies verify that it benefits cancer patients.

ST. JOHN'S WORT

This popular herb may help to alleviate mild depression and has been used for centuries for a wide variety of ailments. Unfortunately, it interferes with a number of medications cancer patients might be taking, such as prescription antidepressants, Digoxin (a heart medicine), Coumadin (a blood thinner), and others. For that reason, it isn't recommended for cancer patients.

BLACK COHOSH

Used to treat hot flashes and menopausal symptoms, this herb is popular in Europe. The root contains phytoestrogens similar to soy products, which could act like natural estrogen in the body. For that reason, it's not recommended for women with breast cancer.

ECHINACEA

An herbal root popular in the United States for two hundred years, echinacea is supposed to enhance the immune system and stimulate white blood cells to help fight cancer. But, like St. John's wort, it can interfere with chemotherapy drugs and, therefore, isn't recommended for breast cancer patients.

ASTRALAGUS

This legume is thought to have immune-enhancing properties. Human studies haven't yet been conducted, so the benefit or risks aren't known.

Whatever choices you investigate to either alleviate some of the side effects of your treatment or to help conquer your cancer, tell your physicians. They need a complete picture of your treatment and can help you to be aware of possible negative combinations of medications.

And be wary of abandoning traditional medicine for alternative methods. I have had patients who did so, including Margaret, who had a lumpectomy with clear margins. Rather than going through chemotherapy, she chose another path, consulting a nutritionist who recommended a strict diet and a regimen of supplements. After a few months, Margaret felt another lump in the same place as the first one. The tumor had recurred quickly, and because of the delay, more aggressive treatment was required to bring the cancer under control.

She immediately came back to me and started chemotherapy.

"I now believe," Margaret said, "if you go to a surgeon, you need to listen to her and follow the protocol."

Margaret's cancer was contained in one breast. She underwent five rounds of chemotherapy, followed by a mastectomy and radiation. Her oncologist recommended a stem cell transplant in which good cells were harvested from Margaret's bone marrow.

"I was in the hospital for a month," she added. "I came as close to dying as I could without actually dying. From that point on I've gotten better. Now I can't tell I've been sick."

Used knowledgeably, herbs, vitamins, and certain foods can bring some relief to nausea and other aspects of your treatment and might help to fight your cancer. If taking these supplements helps you, then you should take them, but never as a replacement for proven medical practices.

Now, on to a closer look at the stress cancer puts on your emotions and how to manage that side of your life in a healthy way.

STRENGTHENING THOUGHTS
FROM GOD'S WORD

"Be strong and courageous. Do not be afraid or terrified . . . , for the Lord your God goes with you; he will never leave you nor forsake you" (Deut. 31:6).

"You have made known to me the path of life" (Ps. 16:11).

"Be strong and take heart, all you who hope in the Lord" (Ps. 31:24).

PART 3

TRAVELING
WITH FINESSE

CHAPTER 10

EMOTIONS: MAKING THEM WORK FOR YOU

Potent emotions come knocking on your door when you learn you have breast cancer. This disease plays no favorites, yields no concessions, refuses bribes, and holds expectations for the future as hostages. Fear, anger, isolation, and despair may insist on moving in and making themselves at home. Questions seem unlimited. How should I react? Do I cry and show emotion or hold it all in to protect others?

How can you take care of yourself emotionally during your journey through breast cancer? How can you toss destructive emotions like fear and despair out the door? What do you do if you're numb and can't pray or just don't know where to look for answers?

The emotions that accompany breast cancer are persistent. You might show them to the door and shove them out, yet they will sneak back in again and again. But you can find ways of thinking that keep you from allowing those emotions to settle in as long-term residents. Let's look at God's wisdom for these circumstances.

BACK TO THE BASICS

Facing cancer takes you straight to your core beliefs—your roots. You learn things about yourself you didn't know. You're offered the opportunity to know your Creator more deeply than ever before. This can be a time of amazing discovery. Although you may not feel your best, your very weakness and need afford God the opportunity to show you tenderness and mercy at a depth you might not have known even existed.

There is no substitute for firsthand experience. It's the difference between reading about training for a battle versus fighting a battle.

To know the Creator, you need to experience him. He alone knows the purpose for your life and when that purpose is fulfilled. He alone knows the number of your days, the path that is yours, and the answers to all the whys. Books or tapes can be helpful, but can't provide all the answers you may be looking for. God is the source of the love, security, and strength that we each need to get through a crisis. He alone really understands. Not even someone who has had a similar experience knows completely how you feel and what you are thinking. God alone saw you before you came into this world, sees how you are growing spiritually, and knows where he wants to take you. His love is personal, specific, and intimate. It has the power to take you to your next step. Nothing else really can. If you try to muster the strength and courage on your own, you may run out of steam before you reach the finish line.

There is much for you to discover in your journey through cancer. First, that real hope is found in God. Cancer is like a spiritual boot camp. You're doing calisthenics designed to strengthen you. You might not have signed up for this, but the opportunity for deep spiritual growth is there as you move through this journey. Look for new spiritual muscles as you exercise your faith.

While experiencing spiritual growth is stimulating and rewarding, that doesn't mean powerful, toxic emotions won't try to settle into your heart. What do you do with them? Let's take a look at the common emotions that accompany you through your breast cancer journey.

ANGER

Emotional recovery is much more complicated than physical recovery; it's a part of breast cancer most women feel least prepared to face. After the initial shock, anger may creep right in and settle down next to you. You might find yourself focusing your anger on the physician who delivered the news, on someone who has been a source of stress in your life, or on a job that hasn't been pleasant.

Anger is part of the grief response associated with serious loss or illness. But a more focused anger might occur as a result of something someone said or did. Any cancer patient can relate a number of such stories. Because of the emotional climate as one fights cancer, little slights or slips of the tongue can become magnified and elicit a strong reaction from you. That doesn't mean the slip, the careless remark, or the insensitive action isn't an offense, but it helps to recognize that your strong reaction is really based in anger and fear about cancer. Redirecting that energy to fighting the cancer can save a relationship and keep the energy from being destructive.

Coping techniques might include talking out the incident with someone, writing about the offense in a letter and then throwing it away, or doing something physical such as a workout. Anger can be productive if it energizes you to fight the cancer; otherwise it works against you. If you are struggling with anger, find a place to get help. Cancer support groups are good launching pads for honest talk. Or discuss your anger with your pastor, a counselor, or a trusted friend.

Anger or disappointment with God may be difficult to admit, but honesty is the first step to healing. Particularly if you're in a position of spiritual leadership, these feelings are disturbing and unwanted, maybe even threatening. But ignoring them or denying them only empowers them. You can dispel much of their power by taking them directly to God.

Margaret came to realize, after her breast cancer diagnosis, "There are worse things in life than cancer—bitterness, unforgiveness, self-absorption, destructive anger, and clinging to our right to a painless life." When she was able to let go of those attitudes, she was freer to fight against the cancer.

For some, anger is not a part of the battle. If that's you, that's great—as long as you're being honest. Perhaps because you've had previous experience with crises or other life events, they prepared you to fight this battle.

FEAR

Anger may be rooted in fear—the fear of losing your life and the fear of what this intruder will mean to relationships, finances, plans, and your own expectations. Once again, you're besieged with questions: What will happen to my children? to my husband? to my marriage?

When Evelyn found out she had cancer, the phone call came when she was alone. "That was my lowest moment," she confessed. "I cried for fifteen minutes. I called my mother, and I was crying so hard she couldn't tell who I was. After I told her the news, my dad, a Baptist minister, got on the phone. He said, 'Get a hold of yourself. Have you forgotten whose you are? You're a child of the King.'" That reminder helped Evelyn to regain perspective and to let go of fear.

"We're scared when we're diagnosed with cancer because we want to live, but it doesn't paralyze us," Margaret said. "I've learned that courage isn't the absence of fear. It's moving forward through fear."

Fear cripples the ability to fight. Conquer fear, and the biggest battle is won. That isn't to minimize the physical aspect of healing, but much of the physical battle will be affected by the mind and the presence or absence of fear.

Ignorance is a great ally of fear. That's why information gathering is so powerful in the beginning of the battle. The idea isn't to overwhelm yourself with information but to garner enough information to develop a working knowledge of the battle and to find answers to your questions. Then engage the enemy and start on your treatment.

Hope helps to defeat fear. Some look to statistics to provide that. They want concrete assurance that they are likely to win this battle. But statistics really come down to what happened to others. They provide a slippery slope of flimsy reassurance. What if the numbers don't look so good? Or if survival is 90 percent, how do you know you aren't part of the 10 percent? Statistics don't offer solid comfort.

As paradoxical as it sounds, fear is overcome when you get sick and then fight through the mental battle of being afraid of illness. Don't run away from the fear; face it and move through it.

Surprisingly, talking about your fear does much to dispel it. This can be a bonding time for you and your loved ones. But it's your job to open that door—no one else is likely to step forward and start the discussion.

Some women work hard to keep their feelings from their families or to avoid talking about death or similar topics in an attempt to protect others. That tact generally has the opposite effect. When you talk about your heart issues, those around you feel relief. They feel they have permission to be honest about how they're feeling and what their fears are.

Spouses and others close to you may experience mental anguish and fear to the same degree you do. When everyone's attention is focused on you, the family might be overlooked, but their pain could be more acute and less addressed than yours. Emotions are high for all concerned, and each family member will most likely be more sensitive during this time. Be especially considerate of each other.

When Jody discovered she had cancer, she made the following resolution: "I don't want to hide the truth about my struggles. Neither do I want them to seem worse than they are. This one thing I know, God is able to keep me. Whether this is light and momentary or heavy and debilitating, he is here beside me."

Just thinking negative thoughts won't make the cancer come back. Nor does thinking positive thoughts prevent the cancer from recurring.

One strategy to defeat fear is to do something fun or stimulating when fear is knocking hard on your front door. Face fear squarely and walk on.

Another practical strategy is to do the opposite of what fear suggests. If you're afraid to do something, do precisely the thing that prompted the fear. If that's too much to handle, take a small step in that direction. Refuse to let fear dictate your behavior.

Psalm 34 teaches us to praise the Lord at all times and to take our troubles to him. That means intentionally to set your mind on him, especially in those times of fear when you feel least able to do so. Even a small step helps. Measure success by taking small steps that put you ahead of where you were yesterday—or an hour ago.

DEPRESSION

Depression is another unwelcome guest that may be heightened or instigated by fear. After surgery, you may feel down for several days or even longer. After gearing up emotionally and physically for the procedure, when it's over, you begin to relax a little and then find yourself facing the new anxiety of chemotherapy and the uncertainty of what the next few weeks will hold. Expect an emotional roller coaster for a few weeks. Physical exhaustion plays into this as well. If you get stuck in a down cycle and can't move through it, talk to your doctor and get professional help.

Antidepressants exist to aid you through times like this. But they aren't the ultimate solution for everyone. Once again, there is no "normal" response; each patient is unique, and what brings resolution to the depression can be different for each person.

JoAnn had struggled with depression on and off for years before being diagnosed with breast cancer. In the weeks following her lumpectomy, anxiety seemed to be dragging her into its merciless grasp. Her primary physician had prescribed medication, which she took, but in spite of that, she laid awake at night, counting the minutes as they crawled by. Longing for the first rays of dawn, she found when they finally broke through the night, there still was no relief from the awful, gnawing anxiety that refused to release its grasp. This continued night after night.

JoAnn and her husband, Dick, both arrived exhausted to a doctor's appointment after driving in the early morning hours trying to relax and break the tension. Sensing that more medication was not the answer, the doctor prayed with them that morning. Dick was as exhausted as his wife, and both sensed immediate relief. He felt the presence of Jesus in that room in a way he hadn't known before. The anxiety was broken at last for JoAnn. She slept well that night and thereafter. Her relationship with Jesus deepened as she learned to lean into his strength in this crisis. Years later, they both look at that moment of prayer as a turning point in their lives.

Making it through your cancer treatment with your spirits intact doesn't mean the battle is over. Once the treatment is complete, you'll go through another transition time and could very likely feel depression or other emotional ups and downs. You realize in more profound ways that breast cancer isn't necessarily a death sentence. Although those words of reassurance might have been said previously, they don't become real until treatment stops and you regain strength physically.

You may begin to explore in more depth the emotional and spiritual impact of the preceding months. The visits to the doctors and the treatments, as unpleasant as they may have been, provided a sense that a battle was being waged on your behalf. The disengagement from all the medical attention is yet one more loss, as odd as that sounds. Now you have to adjust to routine life and cope with not having the medical attention while still resolving the emotions provoked by the cancer.

Family and friends might not understand. In their view, the cancer has been treated, and they're ready to return to a normal life. They encourage you to put this behind you and move on. And they are less sympathetic with your tears.

Women who return to their usual responsibilities without dealing with their emotions may find that months or years later they are hit with depression again. Getting back to other activities is healthy, but it shouldn't be an escape from feelings. Don't pressure yourself to hurry up to return to "normal." Coping with the fear, anger, and depression involves a struggle that can't be avoided, only delayed. Healthy patients are those who can talk about all aspects of their cancer experience, including the struggles, tears, and once unspoken thoughts.

Rest and time will help, but so can someone who has been through a similar experience and can provide understanding.

Support groups and counselors are very helpful. You might feel like being alone, but don't stay there. Often the time you least feel like talking is when you need to talk the most.

And realize that the battle you're fighting is on two planes—the physical and the emotional. As Jody told her friends, "I've never been so tired in my life. I never want to forget what it felt like to be so tired I couldn't read or see. I never want to forget how much patience it takes for someone without physical strength to think properly, what it is like to have no appetite, or how good you need to feel to wear a wig or at least a scarf. God has certainly put me in a wonderful position to realize that I am not my body. But this week I grew tired of playing the patient, long-suffering servant. Oh, how I have struggled with God's plan this week. And yet God remains." Jody's honesty and willingness to talk through her emotional dip will serve her well.

Refuse to let depression control your behavior. Do something fun even when you don't feel like it. And if you have no energy, watch a funny movie or read a humorous book.

Also, looking good can make you feel better. Keep up your personal hygiene and appearance.

GRIEF

Grief is part of the healing process, but no one way to grieve is the correct way. Give yourself permission to experience your losses at your own pace and in your own way. Tears don't need to be explained or justified. Grief can't be denied away or forced into a timetable. The best way to get through it is to accept the process rather than push it away.

Jan Pettigrew is a nurse practitioner who specializes in grief counseling. She has guided hundreds of cancer patients through their grief and teaches them to "lean into it." Denying feelings you don't want only empowers them, and they resurface at a time of their choosing with renewed vigor.

As time elapses, the periods of pain or tears become less frequent and shorter. But in some cases, the real grieving still might hit months or years after cancer. You may not even be aware of denying feelings of anger or grief. You may feel emotional pain, but have a blunted emotional response to everything. You may no longer feel passionate about anything and be unable to laugh or cry. Once recognized, the only solution is to go back and do the grief work you refused to do before.

This can be confusing to the rest of the family. Three years after breast cancer, you might just begin dealing with your emotional pain. Your supporters are likely to feel this is unhealthy and to urge you to "get over it and move on." While the intention is good, this may serve to hinder and to prolong recovery.

In some cases the tears and struggles are not healthy. Patients who aren't recovering well, when asked how they are doing, often become rigid, refuse to have eye contact, and say they are doing fine, but offer no additional comments. If their depression and anger persist many weeks or months without progress or resolution, they become destructive. They need to seek counsel, choose to listen, and make changes.

FINDING SUPPORT

As you work through the emotions of breast cancer, be in touch with friends or family members who can offer support and a safe place to express your emotions. If you have medical decisions still to make or need medical information, turn to your surgeon, primary physician, or other professionals who deal with breast cancer.

Despite good intentions, friends may give erroneous information. If a friend offers counsel or says something you don't find helpful, keep in focus that person's intention of the heart and accept it as a caring gesture while discarding the information.

Some friends and relatives might make comments or express the attitude that, if you ate right and lived right, this wouldn't happen to you. Such thoughts—even if they're your thoughts—can lead to guilt.

"And what about stress?" your friends might ask. "Did you bring this on by living a stressful existence?" Stress may be higher prior to some major medical illnesses, but it's one of many risk factors, not the determining factor.

Such remarks are similar to the ones Job's comforters made. Rather than attempting to comfort Job, his friends were explaining to themselves why his fate wouldn't happen to them—they hadn't done whatever it was Job had done.

Energy directed at trying to figure out why breast cancer happened is wasted energy. While many books and articles claim to understand why a person gets cancer, underlying these explanations is the need to have control. And we don't have control. The reasons for cancer are complex and don't lend themselves to simplistic answers. If need be, decide what you want to attribute it to that isn't self-destructive and leave it there. Pick something so you can move on and use your energy to fight this enemy.

Cancer is a serious battle; the choices are to fight or to surrender. Fighting means facing the problem squarely and honestly, becoming informed, cherishing good days, and making it through bad days, a step at a time.

Jane, whose husband was a pastor, knew her Bible well when diagnosed with breast cancer. She found that cancer deepened her roots in Jesus, but it took time. The passing of several years after the initial diagnosis helped to clarify some of the lessons and growth that came from the experience. During treatment, the first Scripture that really touched her heart was Psalm 46:10, "Be still, and know that I am God." Jane said, "God had to still my life previously to get my focus directed to him. I recognized that when my path and plans were halted this time, I had to be 'still' again and work on my focus. A lot of time I didn't feel like being anything else but still! But then I could see and know God more intimately. His character, his love, his mercy.

"Since I had to be completely dependent on him and to completely trust that he had things in control, I recognized him more readily. He often used my family, friends, and even strangers to meet my physical needs. I couldn't have gotten through day by day without them and their support. But it was so comforting to know that God was in control and to feel his presence completely. That trust will always be with me. I know he can and will be my provision. I can better understand Isaiah 26:3, 'You will keep in perfect peace him whose mind is steadfast, because he trusts in you.'"

YOUR FAMILY'S EMOTIONS

Breast cancer affects the entire family. Your spouse, friends, children, and parents all go through a grieving process. As family members, respect the individual healing process that others go through and give each other time and space. Each person needs room to struggle with questions before God, needs space to be angry, even needs a chance to be unavailable at times. None of these responses indicates an abnormal or unhealthy relationship. They do reflect a normal progression toward healing. No two people follow the same path because each is wonderfully unique.

Caretakers, while suffering equally, might not be excused from performing normal responsibilities. Your spouse's stress might be greater, yet not recognized or addressed. He might be trying to figure out what is the highest priority: his job, which is the source for health insurance, or your illness. His stress might affect his job performance and ability to concentrate there.

Husbands or family may have difficulty facing the reality that they aren't as brave or strong as they would like to think they are. Admonishing them for thinking of themselves instead of you can exacerbate the depression and exhaustion. It leaves them without permission to take care of their own needs and to heal, which ultimately will harm their recovery and usefulness to the family.

Give careful consideration to what is said and how to say something so as not to add stress on anyone. This must be balanced with a desire to stay close and share hearts with one another. Your family and friends who stand by you are expressing great commitment that is neither easy nor inexpensive. Blame can be treacherous; be careful to keep it from taking root.

Rather than trying to avoid conversations about death, let it come out. Listen to every detail with each other. It helps to vent the emotion and to dispel the fear. To hold it in allows it to grow and fester. Although a very difficult topic to discuss, make the effort.

One woman tried to talk with husband about her fear of dying. He was uncomfortable and didn't want to discuss it. He didn't recognize the difference between bringing the issue out in the open so that real healing could occur versus dwelling on death. Not facing the tougher issues together is a lost chance for bonding and intimacy. Just because the topic is uncomfortable, don't dismiss it. You may be surprised at the relief that will prevail once the tough issues are out.

Standing together in a common fight can build strong bonds. Words make or break this interaction. Important decisions need to be made. Fear of making a wrong choice or saying the wrong thing can paralyze progress. Help to alleviate that by deciding ahead of time with each other that mistakes are expected and a sign of normal growth. If a marriage is strained prior to cancer, the couple will need to work harder to handle the circumstances. But many relationships have grown deeper with a challenge like cancer. If both parties are willing to work, much healing and good can come. However, expect it to be hard work.

Discussion about the loss of or change in the breast opens up honesty in the relationship and allows the couple to share the loss and grieve together rather than dealing with it in their own separate ways. These changes do affect each partner, and denying that only gives the loss more power. Your recovery from breast cancer is far more important than the presence of a breast, but that doesn't mean the breast isn't missed. Take comfort and strength from the closeness you enjoy with your partner.

We'll discuss the husband-wife relationship and how breast cancer affects it in chapter 11 and give you information on how to help your children through your breast cancer challenge in chapter 12.

OTHER RELATIONSHIPS

Breast cancer treatments are extensive and can seem to go on forever. Don't go through this alone. Those who have the most difficulty coping are those who isolate themselves. Sometimes patients or families don't take advantage of all their possible support in an effort not to bother someone.

When church friends, family, or other support systems are bypassed, not only is an opportunity missed but loved ones may assume their efforts aren't wanted or needed. Rather than feeling relieved, your friends could feel pushed away. Even if you always have preferred independence, and you aren't in the habit of sharing personal trials with others, this is an opportunity to grow and to try a new perspective. Let others help and see what it does for them and for you.

Friends will sort themselves out quickly. Some whom you haven't been close to might come to the forefront. Others you thought you could count on might disappear. This is all normal, and it helps to expect it. What looks like aloofness or distance from friends often is an expression of their own fear or uncertainty as to what to say. Rather than showing a lack of love or concern for you, they might be fighting their own battles related to your cancer. Some friends will be there in the crisis; others will watch from afar.

Karen made a deliberate choice to include her church friends in her battle with breast cancer. She had known several others in her church who had chosen privacy when diagnosed with serious illness. Some were nearly dead before they let others know. These friends had walked alone through a difficult journey, depriving Karen and others of the opportunity to provide comfort and support. To Karen, this was a missed opportunity to let Christ's body be the body. She decided to be an example of willing vulnerability, letting others support and help her.

This wasn't a comfortable choice for her. As a church staff member and a spiritual leader, receiving was hard for her. But she chose not to hide her weakness, and instead let others walk alongside her. As she openly talked about her treatment and day-to-day battles, others grew comfortable in approaching her.

Support groups allow women to gain strength from one another. Some patients feel such groups were just as important to their recovery as the physical treatment. Consider attending such a group even if you feel you don't need it. Ask for help you don't feel you need. Don't depend on your feelings to let you know.

Support groups come in different varieties. Some are for all types of cancer, some just for breast cancer. Some are primarily informational, others for building support and relationships. All have value, and different types of groups are needed at different times.

Hospitals often have cancer survivor programs and volunteers. Some have hospital chaplains. The American Cancer Society sponsors Reach for Recovery, a volunteer program of women who have recovered from breast cancer.

Counseling can be a safe place to talk out things friends either don't want to hear or don't know how to handle. A counselor may help you to address and control fear as well.

To Work or Not to Work

Continuing to work during treatment helps you to keep your focus off cancer and could result in unexpected expressions of caring from customers or colleagues. If you never talk about your illness with work colleagues or friends, you may end up regretting that decision because of lost opportunities to connect with others. You may be concerned that colleagues will see you as weak because of illness, but in actuality, your battle might very well instill a sense of strength in you for having survived the ordeal. It might open corporate doors rather than close them.

Some have found unexpected support from colleagues that would never have been discovered otherwise. Talking directly with people diminishes speculation and gossip as well as eases tension. The tension arises because people aren't sure what to say or how to say it. They want to express compassion and concern, but don't know how. You break that awkward silence by giving them brief but direct information. Then everyone can move on to the business of the day. If you are in a situation where you may have to give the story fifty times, your strategy might be to designate a close friend as the official contact so you aren't distracted from your work and forced to spend all day talking about breast cancer.

Some women enjoy the time away from work because they've scheduled a variety of fun and stimulating activities. Let this be a time you pamper yourself. Take one day at a time and savor it; find something to enjoy. Enjoy each person who enters your day. Don't fret if you don't feel well or have the energy you are accustomed to having. Accept the limits you have so you can work within them. If you know certain things lift your spirits, such as beautiful music or nature, be intentional about including them in your day.

Whether you return to work as quickly as possible or stay out a few extra days, be kind to yourself. Don't let the cancer control everything in your life; rather make it enhance your life. In general, keeping up your usual activities as much as is reasonable helps to restore order and a sense of normalcy.

As Jody said, when looking back on the tumultuous emotions and physical stresses of her cancer journey, "Sometimes I didn't know if I was hungry or full, sad or glad, weak or strong. Every reference point was missing—except God. He never let me go." For each woman who must make her way through breast cancer and its attending emotions, that really is the point, isn't it? God will remain faithful through anger, fear, depression, and guilt. And his strength will be sufficient even for this journey.

What Loved Ones Can Do

Grief, anger, and depression are to be expected after a cancer diagnosis. Listen first, talk later. Depending on the patient's personality, it may be appropriate to open the conversation with a question or expression of concern so she knows you're willing to talk about how she feels. Listening can be the greatest gift you give a breast cancer patient; that alone can be therapeutic. Refrain from offering medical advice in general. Problem-solving isn't usually what the patient is looking for so much as empathy expressed through just being there.

Listening and caring without advising or solving issues requires more of you in every way. It's more work to truly listen and stay free of judgment or stumbling over the patient's struggles than it is to fall prey to the temptation to demonstrate your wisdom or try to rescue.

Listening well requires great discipline not to judge, question, or even guide. Let the patient work it out and don't hold on to anything said. Letting it pass on through you is what makes it safe for the patient.

If your friend wants to talk about death, let it come out. Listen to every detail. Talking about death helps vent the emotion and dispel the fear. To hold it in allows the fear to grow and fester. Although a very difficult topic to discuss, make the effort. You may find you grow in the process.

Your friend may need to talk about the breast cancer, or she may want to focus on something else. Talk about the same things you talked about before breast cancer. If possible, do the same things together you did before.

One family that decided to have days set aside to be free of talk about cancer found that to be a very successful strategy. Family members screened phone calls and filtered out calls focused on a patient update or anything to do with cancer. Treating a patient as if nothing is different can be very healthy and get the focus off cancer. Be alert and sensitive, however. Your goal is to relieve tension and stress, not seem uninterested in her battle. Relax. Just being you is best.

Sometimes you'll need to cheer up the patient, but compassionate listening is often the first choice among all the responses possible. Comments such as "don't worry," and "you'll do fine" reflect your desire to reassure and comfort, but they can be irritating because they tend to trivialize the emotional pain your friend is in.

And comments that tell the patient what to do risk making you irritating rather than helpful. It's better to simply state what you feel or what you are doing to help, such as, "I want you to know how much I care," "I'm bringing over dinner," or "We would like to take the kids for an afternoon." Give advice only if it's solicited by the patient.

Don't be afraid to cry together. It can help you to bond and help you both to get through the experience.

Honesty and communication need to be emphasized, even overemphasized, because in a crisis, these are more difficult than usual. Express genuine concern and compassion. Don't comment one way or the other on her physical appearance; it just isn't useful.

Watch your words, particularly in stressful times. Your mind might turn to another day when someone else you knew had cancer or another kind of crisis. Before you realize it, you are relaying a horror story. You meant no harm and, in fact, were trying to be empathetic. Clearly these stories are not helpful. Negative words need to be cut off in favor of more positive or encouraging stories.

You may be able to provide a safe place for your friend or her loved ones to talk about relationship changes. If you aren't the right one, you might know who is and be able to provide support and encouragement in seeking out professional resources. Your friend usually needs a safe place to sort through fears and emotions. An outside ear may be helpful even when family relationships are close because loved ones are emotionally involved and healing themselves.

Remember that food preferences might change for the patient, especially during chemotherapy. Try to be flexible and meet your loved one's needs as best you can. And don't forget, for the patient, having friends and family around often is a helpful element of recovery. Be available to spend time with the patient.

Help everyone involved deal with stress. Pay attention to and notice your own responses to stress. Address the source of the stress sooner rather than later. Symptoms of stress include: irritability, fatigue, loss of appetite or overeating, insomnia, difficulty making decisions. For children, rebellion is another expression of stress. Recognize these symptoms for what they are so the underlying cause can be addressed.

One family member might be carrying more of the burden than others realize. Take these symptoms as a clue that communication is needed, then work out the issue. Talking is a first step, but often action is required as well. Eliminate an activity, change a schedule, reassign a responsibility, say no to something. Remember to be reasonable in your expectations of others and be merciful with their shortcomings as well as with your own. Deal with one issue at a time, resolving it before going on to another one.

Don't lose your sense of humor. Look for funny stories or things to laugh about that can help relieve tension. Laughing doesn't make light of an issue; it simply relieves tension so you can address the issue more objectively. Focus on the ultimate message: I care, and you can lean on me.

STRENGTHENING THOUGHTS
FROM GOD'S WORD

"Jesus looked at them and said, 'With man this is impossible, but with God all things are possible'" (Matt. 19:26).

"I will extol the Lord at all times; his praise will always be on my lips" (Ps. 34:1).

"I will lie down and sleep in peace, for you alone, O Lord, make me dwell in safety" (Ps. 4:8).

CHAPTER 11

YOUR SPOUSE, YOUR BIGGEST SUPPORTER

When your husband hears your diagnosis of breast cancer, a pain stabs his heart, just as it does yours. As the reality seeps in, he finds he has the task of being your biggest supporter both emotionally and physically while dealing with his own anxiety and physical stress, and balancing how to help you, yet keep up with his job.

How can the two of you walk through this unfamiliar, uncomfortable territory? How can you come through the journey more of a team and closer to each other than when the trip began? How do you face the challenges so they pull you together rather than apart? What about *his* fears? What about the demands this places on him? And how will cancer affect the emotional and sexual sides of your life together? These are the questions we'll look at in this chapter.

Your husband's consistent presence might well be the greatest gift he can give you during this time. When you feel anxious and are reeling from the news of breast cancer, his quiet presence can reach the deep, hurting places in your heart at a time when words might fall uselessly to the floor.

But the reality is that the two of you might experience different reactions and feelings about the cancer battle. You will each handle stress differently and need different types of support to get you through. As long as that's understood by both of you, you'll enter into this foray with the healthiest asset a couple can have—the willingness to work through each of your concerns, struggles, and fears. The more you share together, the stronger the bond and the more the relationship will grow. Let's take a look at the ways you both need to be willing to let your relationship shift.

CHANGING ROLES

Be aware that changes in the relationship are to be expected. Both of you need to realize that anything as serious as cancer and possible mortality prompts a person to reexamine priorities. The process is healthy and to be welcomed. Good will come from it.

A woman who has enjoyed being taken care of might decide she now wants to make more decisions. Her husband might not see why this change is important for her or might feel threatened in the relationship. His attitude could discourage her progress. The pleasant surprise is that if a husband can allow and even encourage the changes, both will find the relationship deeper, more satisfying, and more stimulating.

If you have always been the one to take care of everything, now you might like to be taken care of, even if it's for just a few weeks. Once again, this might feel strange to both of you and not be understood as a healthy process. But if your husband can accept the change and take on the role of protector and decision-maker, the relationship will deepen and become healthier. But you both need to talk about this shift in your relationship and give each other time to adjust.

If the changes that occur in your relationship can be welcomed and each partner is allowed to grow and try different roles, it will ultimately improve the relationship and build stability, although that might not be apparent initially. Humor can help to break the tension from the expected misunderstandings that go along with growth. Grab for humor wherever you can find it, and even in the midst of cancer, try not to take yourself too seriously.

Your friends and family can be overprotective or too inattentive. Expect to make adjustments along the way according to what you learn about yourself. And remember that only when you tell your loved ones what you need can they know how to respond. Don't expect your husband to be a mind reader, especially during this time in which you are encountering challenges and fears you've never had to face before. And let your husband know whether you want family or friends around when you are feeling ill. Most women prefer only one or two helpers at these times.

ADJUSTING HOUSEHOLD ROLES

Adapt to new household duties, if necessary. Nurture and cultivate a mutual trust and respect for one another rather than for the roles you've played in the past. Let the challenge of illness pull you together as a team. This must be intentional. Without specific attention, relationships tend to drift apart anyway, but under the added pressures of fighting cancer, it takes all the more work to talk through each other's insecurities, worries, and fears. Cancer requires even more diligence to keep open the lines of communication, cooperation, and trust.

Nothing is more heartrending than to see couples who encounter cancer and try to shield each other from their emotions.

They mean well. Because they care about their spouse, they are trying to protect the other person from deep emotional pain, and they are trying to be strong. While the intention is good, the outcome is tragic. Instead of sparing the person pain, they are instead creating an invisible wedge. Much greater than the pain of those disturbing feelings they would rather not admit is the pain of distance growing in the relationship. Now, instead of a couple pooling their insight and emotional energy for a stronger whole, they are each fighting separately.

The Sexual Side of the Relationship

When you come home from the hospital, you and your husband won't be entirely sure how physical each of you will want to be. Communicate with one another. Most women at that point desperately need a touch, an assurance that they are still attractive to their husbands. If your husband backs off, he might be trying to show you consideration until you feel stronger, but you might interpret his physical distance incorrectly. That's why you need to talk about it.

Some couples are intimate with each other within hours after arriving home from the hospital with no problems. Others prefer affection with abstention for a while until she feels stronger. No formula exists for this time, but whatever choices you make will set the tone for the relationship, at least for the time being. There is no substitute for communicating.

This is a great time to lavish reassurances of love and attractiveness on each other. While you might feel fatigued and perhaps unattractive, let your husband know you need encouragement. Let him know that his words can help to assuage sensitive areas in your heart. And help him to understand that if you negate his words, it's highly likely you're signaling that you need further affirmation and encouragement.

One young wife felt this way: "The idea of sexual relations after surgery was just one more stress. How would my husband react? We rarely had sexual relationships without him reaching for my breasts. How was he going to feel with one missing? I needed to feel close to him. I needed to know I still aroused him. So the night I got home from the hospital we made love. I concealed my breasts from him not only that night, but also for seven more days. That was a big mistake. He didn't push me to show him. But I began to wish he would press to see the scar, because my fear of revealing myself was growing.

"Looking back now, I should have shown him the surgery site in the hospital. Worrying for over a week caused self-inflicted, unnecessary stress. The relief I felt the morning I showed him was so welcome. And my fears were unfounded. He calmly assured me the scar was about what he thought it would look like. He told me he loved me, and that he was glad of my decision. Then he held me in his arms, saying nothing, while I cried. Sometimes the best thing to say is nothing. He didn't try to tell me it was going to be all right or not to cry; instead, he did the best thing ever by just being there and letting my emotions flow."

As a couple, talk about when your husband should see the surgical incisions. Some couples decide they will see the incision together for the first time. Others might prefer to handle it differently. Once again, the key is communication and support. Your husband might want to touch the surgery site once it's healed. Some women don't like their husbands to touch it. But most find it draws them together and helps her to adjust. And your husband might massage the surgical site to help alleviate phantom pain or discomfort for you.

"I think all women are worried about whether they will be able to arouse their husbands in bed," one husband of a patient in her early thirties said. "They worry that he will be turned off by the loss of a breast. That's the woman's view, not the man's. It wasn't my view. The absence of a breast didn't matter in the sexual relationship."

Talk over with your husband how you feel about your missing breast and give him the opportunity to do the same. This is a good place to begin honest discussion that allows you both to share the grief. The loss of a breast does touch each partner, and denying that only gives the loss more power over you. Your husband cares far more about your recovery from breast cancer than he does about the presence of a breast. But that doesn't mean the breast isn't missed. It is. Take that sense of loss to the Lord. And don't turn away from each other.

YOUR HUSBAND'S NEEDS

Husbands can attempt to use their analytical and problem-solving skills for you. Although that's natural, be honest if you would rather he simply listen and not offer possible solutions. Tell him what you need that would communicate his love to you. Try to look for what helps him as well.

Ask your husband questions that give him the opportunity to talk about his feelings. But don't push; just provide an open attitude and a listening ear. Healing begins when you both can admit what you're feeling and realize these responses are normal.

Either or both of you might feel resentful that this has happened. Cancer has interrupted all your plans. It has brought fear, inconvenience, and pain. While your husband knows you didn't intentionally get cancer, a corner of his heart might feel anger with you for causing this stress and disrupting the family. As an adult, he sees how ridiculous that thought is, but that idea doesn't need to have any basis in reality or logic to lodge in his mind. He can't make the emotion go away by telling himself what a silly, selfish thought that is.

Your husband might want to talk out his feelings with a trusted friend, pastor, counselor, or with you. Be open to his turning to someone else to talk about his negative emotions. He needs room to make those choices, just as you do. Once these feelings are faced and brought out in the open, the power of that annoying thought is broken. It evaporates, and you both can expend your energy dealing with what is real.

One way for either of you to determine what you need to deal with is to hone in on any thought or feeling that makes you feel guilty. That thought is an energy robber, and admitting it deals it a lethal blow.

Some families can talk to each other about these very real feelings; others have never learned to do so. Some family members would experience hurt feelings if these things came out in a discussion. The solution will be different in every home. If you aren't accustomed to talking at this level, a counselor or close friend might be a better place to take the emotions. But an intimacy and closeness results from being able to face these emotions together as a couple. It takes a maturity that recognizes the other person is not attacking but rather confessing thoughts and feelings so they can be dispersed and evaporate.

Ed was in his early thirties when his wife was diagnosed with breast cancer. He admits now, several years later, that he didn't cope well with the diagnosis. He didn't talk with his wife about anything to do with her breast cancer. Although he knew that she was the same attractive person she had always been, emotionally he shut down.

Denial was his initial coping mechanism. Ed said, "I went into the mode of deciding everything would be okay. She will get through it, and her mom and dad are there to support her. I've got to go to work, and I'll just go on with my everyday normal routine. Everything will be fine."

Denial can offer some protection while the shock and pain are acute and coping abilities undeveloped. For Ed, renewing his relationship with Christ was a key to finding the strength to face his wife's cancer. His wife also turned to Christ as her source of strength during this battle with breast cancer. Ed regrets his initial lack of support for her, but with God in his life, he is making progress toward healing the hurting places in his own heart. They now are able to discuss the cancer and other sensitive issues.

Each couple must find their own way through breast cancer. But the common elements of communication and sensitivity to the unique healing process for each family member paves the way for stronger relationships. In the next chapter, we will look at children's needs during this stressful time in a family's life.

WHAT LOVED ONES CAN DO

Family members and friends need to realize that support for men may look different than that for women. Instead of talking, men might find doing something with a friend is the type of support they find most effective. Let activities begin the healing process, but don't let it stop there. Precisely because men don't open up easily, they may need help with that from other caring men. A pastor, male counselor, or close male friend can be a significant help. Ask specific questions such as, "Are you sleeping okay?" "Are you going to work?" "Could I join you when you visit your wife tomorrow?" Offer specific help: Take him out to dinner. Ask if he would like to play a round of golf with you. Send him a card.

STRENGTHENING THOUGHTS
FROM GOD'S WORD

"Love covers over all wrongs" (Prov. 10:12).

"Better a meal of vegetables where there is love than a fattened calf with hatred" (Prov. 15:17).

"Like an apple tree among the trees of the forest is my lover among the young men. I delight to sit in his shade, and his fruit is sweet to my taste. He has taken me to the banquet hall, and his banner over me is love" (Song 2:34).

CHAPTER 12

HELPING CHILDREN FACE THE CHALLENGE

Once a mother begins to absorb the shock of being told she has breast cancer, one of her immediate responses is to think about how her children will face this crisis. Ultimately, if you allow your children to be a part of your healing process, everyone—you and your children—will fare better. Once they understand that you will share honestly with them about your treatment and what it means, they feel more secure. Your openness gives them permission to ask questions that you would never have anticipated they were thinking.

Children react differently to the news of their mother's breast cancer according to their age and maturity as well as their unique personalities. Small children will reflect their parents' emotional tone. If you're positive and upbeat in explaining what will happen, they will be as well. If you're fearful and negative, they will reflect that.

A parent's cancer disrupts a child's world and may lead to fear and insecurity. Children often feel angry and perhaps abandoned or guilty. Although they did nothing to cause your cancer, and they are not being abandoned, still the emotions are present. Overt anger, rebellion, poor performance at school, irritability, and significant change in behavior can signal you that your child needs compassion and help in dealing with these unwanted emotions.

Look for the root cause. Help your children to vent and to admit the feelings. Then provide lots of acceptance and love. Teach them that although the feelings are very real, they are not valid. Scolding or punishing can make the underlying depression or fear worse. Extra love, reassurance, and acceptance may help your child feel more secure. Emphasize to the child that he or she didn't cause the cancer and won't be abandoned. Regularly reinforce that you are not sick because of something your children said or did.

Breaking the News

The best time to discuss cancer and the upcoming events associated with it is as soon as you feel emotionally under control. Children quickly sense when something is up and know if they are being excluded from a significant event. This fosters insecurity. Since their natural tendency is to imagine the worst, the sooner parents dispel that, the better. If a medical crisis occurs, the children will respond best if information is shared as problems arise. Ignorance makes kids more vulnerable and allows for misconceptions. Also, keep in mind that children take pride in helping and being involved. Deliberately look for ways they can participate and help.

What to tell your child will depend on his or her personality and maturity level. Cover briefly but clearly the things that directly affect his world. Explain what you have, how it will be treated, and what that means for the child for the next few weeks. Explain that it's not contagious, like other illnesses they might be more familiar with. Allow them to ask for further information when and if they want it. You don't need to cover every detail of treatment or your anxiety in waiting for test results to come back.

Children need to know that their physical and emotional needs will be met. Young children live in a self-centered world. That's part of their very normal immaturity. Don't require them to be adults in their attitudes and behavior. Although your needs may be far more acute, reassure them that their needs will be met. It's fine if they see you tearful at times, but don't look to them for the emotional support you need.

Keep their routines as normal as possible. If they are involved in sports or other extracurricular activities, ask friends to provide rides or attend the events in your place. If you lack the energy to plan birthday parties, ask a friend or family member. And if celebrations need to be postponed, reschedule them with the child, putting the new dates on the calendar together.

HELPING YOUR TEEN

Teenagers may turn more to their peers for support. Although this is normal and expected, peers may not have the answers your child needs. Make teachers, youth workers, and other adults who have relationships with your children aware of your circumstances. Perhaps it isn't your style to ask for help or to divulge personal information to teachers or school counselors. But these people usually are more than willing to offer help and support if you allow them to do so, and it could be critical for your child. That teacher or youth worker may be in a strategic place to see or observe something you would never know about and can intervene.

DEALING WITH NEW BEHAVIOR

If you're having difficulty determining the cause of unwanted, new behavior, stop and deal with that issue—and that issue only—the next time it occurs. Don't try to deal with the whole spectrum of behavior. See if the child will open up and give you a clue as to what feelings or fears are behind this one incident.

Don't allow one child's issues to control the entire family. Seek professional counseling if behavioral issues aren't resolving. Just as your emotions can catch up with you a year or two after your cancer diagnosis, the same could be true of your children's reactions. Kids might gear up emotionally for the immediate challenge of Mom's breast cancer, then experience spiritual or emotional battles later. Typically a change in behavior is the tip-off.

LEARNING ABOUT LIFE

Children are learning appropriate ways to handle their own stress and emotions by watching how you handle cancer. Work intentionally on rapport and communication with each child. This is harder when you don't feel well, but a little goes further than you might expect. Encourage them to vent feelings of anger, fear, or resentment and use the opportunity to teach them when and how it is appropriate to do so. Give yourself some breathing room when you need it and don't feel guilty if you can't always be there for your kids. Your best is good enough.

Your kids will be watching intently as you handle this crisis, and what you do will prepare them for crises in their own lives in the future. Details are important. Do you and your spouse continue to show respect and love for one another? Are mistakes okay? How do you handle them? For instance, if you are tired and cranky and yell at the kids, do you apologize and assure them of your love? No parent does everything right all the time, and parenting is extra hard when you don't feel well. Just be aware that little things you hardly notice may have a big impact on your children. Communication on their level is extra important at this time. And expect a few surprises in their responses.

Here is one young mother's story of an incident with her child:

"Twenty days after my first treatment, the tingling of my scalp and the shedding of my hair all over my pillow announced that my hair would soon be history. *How could I delay this?* I thought. Sure, I had the wig and assorted turbans, but mentally I needed a little more time. My solution was not to wash my hair for two days (causing yet more worry trying to prolong the inevitable!). But I think God used that stalling tactic in his own unique way.

"The day after my second treatment, only my four-year-old son, Jared, was home with me, watching TV in the den. Needing to be alone for this next difficult step, I went to our bathroom, laid my wig on the counter, and stepped into the shower. Just as I thought, all of my hair was soon lying on the shower floor. As I stepped out of the shower, the sobs that had been building within for so long erupted. I cried long and hard. My stomach hurt. I had had several little cries over the last two months, but this was the one I needed.

"Through my tears, I heard my son crying behind me. The mother in me quickly forgot my hair and was concerned with what would cause my precious boy to cry. I asked Jared if he was hurt.

"He said no.

"'Why are you crying?'

"'I'm sorry.'

"'Did you break something or hurt the new kitten?'

"He again shook his head no and just said he was sorry.

"'Sorry for what?' I asked.

"'I don't know, but it must have been really bad since you're mad enough to pull your hair out.'

"I laughed—and I mean roaring laughter. I gathered Jared in my arms and let him touch my head. I explained to him how 'Big Red' (what we called the chemotherapy) was running around in my body killing all bad cells that grow fast. I explained that my hair cells grew fast and that Red couldn't tell the difference.

"He asked with a big smile on his face, 'So it's doing its job, killing the cancer?'

"Then it hit me like a ray of sunshine. 'You know, son, we had no way of knowing if it was working until today, but if it can kill my hair, the medicine can destroy any cancer left in my body.'

"'Mom, I'm glad you no longer have cancer.' Then he slid off my lap and disappeared to watch TV again with a big smile on his face.

"I turned around, stared in the mirror, and smiled, too. Who would have thought that explaining to my four-year-old that losing my hair was the only sign I had that the drugs were working had just explained it to me. The chemotherapy was working in my body. From that day on, every time I looked in the mirror I smiled."

Although cancer represents a tremendous stress to any family, it also creates powerful teaching moments. Recognize those moments, and in spite of your being weak and not at your best, remember that your actions and words will carry greater impact than usual.

Cindy Brinker Simmons was a young child as she watched her mother, tennis star Maureen Connolly Brinker, struggle through ovarian cancer that eventually claimed her life.

At the age of nineteen, Maureen was the world tennis champion. Her career ended abruptly when she tore tendons her leg in a freak accident. "[There was] no railing against fate, no cursing the unfairness of it, just a clear-eyed realization that this was probably the end [of her tennis career]," Cindy said.

"Mom exhibited an attitude of gratitude for what tennis had done for her, the places she had been, and the people she had met. There was no room for self-pity. Instead, she chose joy. She accepted the present and looked forward to the future instead of looking back at the past. She was at peace with her circumstances and chose to greet each new day with a smile.

"Many times, circumstances have been beyond my control, but my responses to those circumstances are something I can control. Mom was so gracious and positive, even in dying, that her example would not allow me to be bitter.

"Why? Because Mom dealt with dying the same way she dealt with living: by embracing it, by being strong, by being positive, by facing her fear with courage, by strategizing her road to victory and, most importantly, doing all of this in a humble manner. She would have been so disappointed if she thought that through her death I was grieving to the point of being immobilized or angry beyond reason."[1]

Cindy's mother's attitude continues to have a powerful effect on her daughter and on many others her life touched. A big part of the impact was a result of people watching her handle the battle with ovarian cancer. She refused to allow the cancer to control her. Rather, she controlled it by her attitude and positive influence on others. The same can be true for you. Love your children, listen to them as they struggle to face this crisis with you, and let them see you make your way through your cancer journey with all the strength and courage you can muster. It will make a world of difference for them.

WHAT LOVED ONES CAN DO

Friends that can be attentive to the emotional support for the family are helping the patient as well. When offering help, be thoughtful, creative, and specific.

Suggestions might be to help with transportation, pick up items at the grocery store (or take the patient), take the kids to something fun, give the primary caretaker a break and sit with the patient. Close friends may be able to care for the kids during hospitalization, freeing the spouse to be with his wife. Remember that extra expenses such as parking fees, meals out, babysitters, and the like do add up. If you aren't a cook, perhaps a catered meal would be appreciated. Offer to stay and eat with the family and don't be offended if they decline. If your offer of help is not accepted, don't be put off by that. Call again in a few days.

STRENGTHENING THOUGHTS FROM GOD'S WORD

"God sets the lonely in families" (Ps. 68:6).

"As a father has compassion on his children, so the Lord has compassion on those who fear him" (Ps. 103:13).

"May you live to see your children's children" (Ps. 128:6).

CHAPTER 13

RESTORING FITNESS
AND WELL-BEING

After the diagnosis, after the treatment, when at last those stopovers on your journey are in the past, I hope you'll take time to celebrate. You've come through a lot, and you deserve some confetti tossing. You've discovered you're more resilient, braver, and able to do and endure more than you had ever dreamed. And you've learned that when you don't feel brave, resilient, or courageous, you just take the next small step. So, by all means, celebrate, even if it's a small event. Buy yourself a new dress, go to high tea with a best friend, or just settle on the couch with your husband and watch a favorite video.

But be aware that, when treatment is complete, you might very well feel uncomfortable that the medical attention is over. Since no one promises a cure, every ache at this point causes anxiety. Could it mean the cancer is recurring? Or that a complication has set in?

You may feel anxious about not seeing your doctors as often, unsure of what the future holds, still making some significant adjustments to the new you. As much as you want life to get back to what it was before cancer, you are a changed person. For many, the year after cancer treatment is as hard or harder emotionally than the months of treatment. You might not have expected that.

Life and routines begin to move back toward normal. This makes for another transition period, complete with its own set of challenges. Are your loved ones wanting to celebrate? That certainly seems positive and the right idea, but you may feel exhausted from the months of treatment you geared up emotionally to handle.

The exhaustion may take many months to resolve. Most women feel that it takes up to two years after treatment before they feel physically back to normal.

REGAINING SPIRITUAL FITNESS

Are you going through a period of wrestling with God? During treatment, it was all you could do to hang on to his hand, or to let him carry you. Maybe you felt that he was nowhere near. Now questions might surface that you're uncomfortable with or that you prefer not to admit to yourself. Questions like, "How could God let this happen to me?" "What is the purpose for my suffering?" "Why wasn't I healed miraculously?" We discussed those issues in chapter 4, but you might want to revisit that chapter when those pesky questions pop up again.

As I've stated throughout this book, asking tough questions might be uncomfortable, but questioning can be a very healthy process. Don't ignore the questions or feel guilty about them. Take them to God. If you don't know how to do that, look for a pastor or Bible-based counselor to help. Don't try to sidestep the wrestling; rather move into it.

REGAINING PHYSICAL FITNESS

Women who are physically active prior to breast cancer treatment may cut back or eliminate their exercise routines at the initiation of cancer therapy. Stress and fatigue play a big role in that, but research shows that exercise can be very helpful during treatment. Although treatment will necessitate a less rigorous exercise schedule than prior to treatment, often some level of physical conditioning can be maintained. This is especially true for women who exercised regularly before the onset of cancer. As a matter of fact, moderate exercise tends to reduce cancer-related fatigue. However, in some instances exercise might not be recommended, so before beginning any program, make sure you check with your physicians and obtain their approval.

You may feel as though all eyes are on you when you first go out in public after surgery or after hair loss. Although it feels that way, it usually isn't true. And remember, as you head to the gym for your workout, most women you'll meet there are more concerned about their own flaws than looking for flaws in you.

REGAINING EMOTIONAL FITNESS

It's normal to think that every ache or pain might be the cancer coming back, especially in the first few months after treatment. Waves of fear can hit out of nowhere. The fear occurs less frequently with time. If the symptom persists for a couple of weeks or more, see your doctor. If you've lost sleep over it, call your doctor or oncology nurse rather than allow it to continue to terrorize you. He or she can help sort out whether it's anything to be concerned about; one phone call might lay the whole issue to rest, allowing you to conquer the fear and move on. Don't be embarrassed or feel silly when these symptoms surface. They're to be expected after cancer.

If a problem is detected, even if on further testing it turns out to be nothing, the emotional response is often much greater than was typical prior to having cancer. Again, this is normal and expected. Take things one day at a time and don't jump to conclusions. Complete the necessary tests and refuse to let your mind dwell on the negative. Most of the time you will get good answers and the extra tests were just an effort by your physicians to be appropriately cautious.

Jody was ready to get back into exercising after her treatments and had created a plan to walk some days and swim others. But then she developed pain in her hip that caused her to limp even after just sitting for a while. Putting her exercise program on hold, she had X-rays and a bone scan. Of course she feared that the cancer may have traveled to her hip bone, even though she know that was highly unlikely. The tests revealed mild arthritis, and Jody had to set aside her plans for more aggressive exercising.

So she began to explore another avenue of expression that she had avoided in her pre-cancer days. Even though she was an art minor, she never liked any of her own paintings, probably because she compared them to ones by her professional artist mother. But when Jody's exercise program was delayed, she pulled out her brushes and paints and set to work. How had the cancer changed her, enabling her to do what she always wanted to do? "I know it has something to do with realizing in yet a different way what God taught me back at the beginning of my cancer odyssey: that he loves me just as I am."

GETTING PREPARED FOR CHECKUPS

Going in for routine checkups after your treatment is complete can be anxiety producing. The fear lurks that something may be found. Try combating it by doing something fun the night before or perhaps in the morning before the appointment.

The schedule of checkups and tests you will have vary according to your specific situation and your doctor's preferences. In general, you will be followed for at least five years by your medical oncologist and surgeon, and sometimes by the radiation oncologist as well. In some communities the primary physician will do the follow-up after cancer treatment is complete. Lumpectomy patients will have a mammogram of the affected breast every six months. All breast cancer patients will have a mammogram annually. Blood work may be done twice a year. Women on Tamoxifen should have an annual pelvic exam unless the uterus has been removed. A bone density test, different from a bone scan, is appropriate every two or three years to check for osteoporosis. This can be a problem after breast cancer because you won't be taking estrogen. If you aren't sure of what your particular schedule will be, don't hesitate to ask your doctor.

GETTING FIT WITH NUTRITION

Numerous studies have documented decreased cancer incidence in people who eat diets high in fruits, vegetables, and fiber and low in fat. The benefit is thought to be the antioxidants and potentially other less recognized nutrients provided by these foods. These plant chemical compounds, called "phytochemicals," are an area of increasing research. Cruciferous vegetables such as cabbage, brussels sprouts, and broccoli may have phytochemicals that promote less active forms of estrogen, which might benefit breast cancer patients.

High fiber diets have been associated with a slight decrease in breast cancer incidence. Whether increasing dietary fiber after a cancer diagnosis means less possibility of recurrence isn't known. But high fiber diets are beneficial in many respects, so starting or maintaining a high fiber diet won't hurt.

Lifestyle changes that occur gradually and incrementally may be more successful than drastic changes, particularly when the dietary changes seem less palatable than your previous diet. A diet high in fruits, vegetables, and fiber should be just as palatable, but it may take more time to prepare than readily available fast food.

Megadoses of vitamins or other supplements may be counter-productive. Studies indicate a balance of nutrients might work together to promote health better than any single nutrient. Research is ongoing in this area and understanding the complex relationships among nutrients is just beginning. Studies do show that an excessive intake of a single nutrient may increase the risk of cancer. For these reasons, dietary programs using whole foods rather than isolated nutrients are recommended.

SEXUALITY

Any serious illness disrupts your sexual relationship temporarily, but breast cancer adds to the number of potential problems. The emotional impact of losing a breast or the changes in the breast from lumpectomy may affect your confidence or self-esteem. You will likely regain that confidence in time, particularly with a supportive partner who is sensitive to your needs. We address these issues in more depth in chapter 11.

Decreased libido can result from the fatigue, from premature menopause brought on by chemotherapy, and from the stress of treatment and recovery. Vaginal dryness can also contribute to painful intercourse. Vaginal lubricants such as Replens and Astroglide are very helpful when used regularly. Other products such as Estring and VagiFem contain estrogen, but are considered safe because they work topically and are thought to have minimal absorption through the vagina. However, it's best to check with your oncologist before using any estrogen product.

Hot flashes may be difficult to eliminate. Vitamin E was thought to offer some benefit, but research to date hasn't documented fewer hot flashes in women taking vitamin E. Natural estrogen-like compounds found in plant sources such as soy (phytoestrogens) may offer some benefit, but their safety for women who have had breast cancer is uncertain and therefore not currently recommended. A number of antidepressant medications and a blood pressure medication help with hot flashes and may be recommended by your primary physician or oncologist if symptoms warrant. Fortunately hot flashes generally diminish with time.

DEALING WITH LYMPHEDEMA

When lymph nodes are removed under the arm (axillary dissection), the lymphatic channels may not be as efficient in their function, resulting in arm swelling. While this may happen within the first few weeks after surgery, more often it occurs months or years later in around 20 percent of women who have had an axillary dissection. With the newer sentinel node biopsy, far fewer women are likely to experience this swelling.

Initially, the swelling may come and go. Frequently, women can relate their first episode of swelling to something they did, such as heavy lifting or a cut that got infected in the hand or arm. The lymphatic channels are tiny vessels like the blood capillaries and are found throughout the body. These vessels carry fluid that is packed with specialized cells, called lymphocytes, and many other substances that bathe the cells continuously to help fight infections.

Lymph nodes are the bean-shaped structures we have mentioned before. They contain millions of the lymphocytes and other cells in an organized structure. Hundreds, perhaps thousands, of lymph nodes function to protect the body from all sorts of would-be invaders.

The lymphatic channels that previously connected to the removed lymph nodes must reroute the fluid they carry. The body is designed so well that this usually occurs without you even noticing. But for a variety of reasons, that may not always happen perfectly. It is much like a freeway with three lanes in one direction. Suppose one lane gets blocked. That doesn't pose a problem if traffic is light. But if traffic is heavy, then a backup of cars begins to occur. The heavier the traffic, the worse the backup. Swelling in the arm occurs when the lymphatic fluid is "backed up" and the channels can't carry all the fluid necessary.

Heavy lifting often creates this backup because the work that the muscles in the arm are doing stimulates an increased flow of the lymphatic fluid. That increase may be too much for the remaining channels, resulting in swelling. Infection may also result in swelling because part of the body's response to infection is to greatly increase the lymphatic flow to the affected area.

This swelling is usually temporary at first. When the stimulus that increased the flow stops (you stop lifting heavy boxes), the swelling goes down. The swelling may become permanent in time. The reasons for this aren't clear, but if something over the years further reduces the number or efficiency of the outflow channels, your body might be unable to keep up with the lymphatic fluid volume even at rest, and the hand or arm may have permanent swelling. Infections that may damage some of these tiny lymphatic vessels could cause them to close. Also, with aging, perhaps these vessels become less pliable or less able to repair minor breaks.

STEPS TO TAKE FOR SWELLING

1. Stop what you were doing. We do know that the first time you experience swelling, you should stop and determine what seems to be the cause. Were you lifting heavy objects, doing a new exercise involving your arms, flying in an airplane, or fighting an infection in the arm?

2. *Call your physician.* If there is redness or pain in the arm and therefore the possibility of an infection, call your physician and get started on an antibiotic. You can call your surgeon, medical oncologist, or primary physician. If you're several years out from your breast cancer and no longer seeing the surgeon, your primary care physician might be your best choice.

As Jane observes from her own experience and from that of other cancer survivors, "With breast cancer the lymph node removal leaves a numb armpit, but more significantly your immune system in the arm of the affected side could be compromised. For some women, this means that you have to be extremely careful of the arm. Something that would normally be a minor problem can cause a major infection that requires hospitalization. I have a friend who was in the hospital a week from an infected hangnail and another from a mosquito bite. A simple paper cut needs to be treated with antibiotic ointment."

3. *Start taking antibiotics immediately.* Prompt attention and starting on antibiotics right away are important if there is infection in the arm or hand. Because the lymphatic fluid is rich in nutrients, if it is backed up in the arm, that helps the bacteria to grow. When the outflow is slowed, the body can't fight infection as effectively. Infection can spread rapidly and become serious quickly, resulting in hospitalization for IV antibiotics. If you have had one or two episodes of infection in your affected arm, it might be wise to have a prescription for an antibiotic that you can fill at the first sign of another infection. If you're traveling, particularly overseas, you may want to take some antibiotics with you in case they are needed.

Most cuts and scrapes on the affected arm don't become infected. Many times women who have had no problems with the arm feel anxious anytime they get a slight cut or minor injury to the hand or arm. Usually, no special attention is needed. An antibiotic ointment might be used once or twice. Infection that needs attention is obvious: redness and pain beyond just the immediate area of the cut or bite. When in doubt, check with your doctor.

4. *After-surgery treatment.* Opinions vary widely regarding what to do with the affected arm after surgery when no swelling exists. Most physicians recommend the arm be protected by doing blood pressure checks and drawing blood elsewhere, such as on the other arm. The theory behind this is that minimizing the number of skin breaks helps to minimize the potential for infection. The blood pressure cuff could squeeze and damage some of the lymphatic vessels, and avoiding that is useful.

5. *Lose weight.* Weight reduction may be important if you are overweight. The extra burden put on the lymph vessels by the excess weight could be enough to start a problem with lymphedema. Some women have shed pounds and found that reduction in weight significantly reduced swelling in the arm.

In general, I recommend that you treat the surgical arm like you did before surgery. You can carry the same things, push, pull, and, for the most part, pay no special attention. Too often women become overly protective of the arm, fearful that a slight cut is going to result in swelling or infection. In some cases, their whole lifestyle changes, and they become focused on the arm.

6. *Elevate the arm.* Arm elevation is the first step when minimal swelling is noted. If you get your elbow above your heart level, gravity helps move the fluid out of the arm. You can also gently squeeze a rubber ball. That causes the arm muscles to act as a pump that moves the fluid along. This is best done with the arm up as well. For elevation to be effective, you need to rest the arm in that position for at least a couple of hours, longer if possible. That means you

need to cushion the arm on a pillow while sitting and reading or watching TV. Active lifestyles often make this impractical, but it's a good step when feasible.

7. *Buy a custom-made sleeve.* Another step is to be fitted for a sleeve. These are compression garments that are custom made for you. Your doctor can give you a prescription that you take to a shop that carries these garments, where you are measured and the sleeve is ordered. You can wear the sleeve part of the day, while flying, or all day, depending on the need. If you have a lot of swelling, you may want to be remeasured after some of the swelling is reduced so that the garment won't be too large. Some doctors recommend that you wear a sleeve anytime you fly. That's because the air pressure is slightly diminished in the cabin during air travel, and that reduced pressure could result in swelling in your arm. I don't recommend that for women who aren't experiencing swelling in their arms. But once swelling occurs, either temporary or prolonged, this is a good recommendation.

8. *Get a specialized massage.* If these simple measures don't suffice, you could also explore manual lymphatic drainage (MLD). This is a specialized massage technique that originated in Europe and has become popular in the United States. This is not taught as a part of routine massage training or physical therapy training but requires specialized courses, and the therapist becomes certified to do this properly. This massage helps to mobilize fluid out of the affected arm. Usually this is done when women have chronic lymphedema, meaning the swelling in the arm has persisted beyond a few days or weeks. Scheduling the massage can be inconvenient because ideally it is done five days a week for three or four weeks. The arm is wrapped with compression bandages between sessions to maintain the progress made during the session, with gradual improvement over several days.

9. Use a sequential pump. Another option for treating chronic lymphedema is a sequential pump. This is something you can purchase and have available anytime you need to use it. It consists of a plastic tubular sleeve that has air pockets that inflate and deflate sequentially, moving fluid up and out of the arm. It is important to use the sequential pump properly at very low pressures because the lymphatic system is a low-pressure system of vessels. If the pump is used at high pressures (over 30 mmHg), instead of pumping out fluid, the pump can compress and damage lymphatic vessels, eventually making the swelling worse. To be effective, most women will wear the pump for at least two to four hours several times a week. While this is more convenient than going to the MLD therapist, it may not be as effective because of variations in the pressure applied to the arm. Some metropolitan areas have lymphedema clinics where both certified MLD therapists and compression pumps are available.

10. Don't use diuretics. The fluid causing the swelling in lymphedema has a high protein content. Fluid pills (diuretics) that you or others you know may take for occasional swelling or fluid retention don't help the lymphedema and may make it worse. A number of drugs are being studied outside the United States that may increase the breakdown of the protein and help decrease the fluid retention, but none is currently available here.

GIVING BACK

Many patients have discovered that an important part of recovery is helping others along the same path. Giving of yourself and sharing about your experience provide you with a sense of having benefited from your battle with cancer. You'll meet some wonderful fellow cancer survivors as a result.

Ann began a ministry to other breast cancer survivors after being successfully treated. She found that opportunities to speak publicly were coming her way, and from that, she began to communicate with women she had met via email. She would keep track of when they were going in for their chemotherapy or other treatment and provide specific prayer and support at the most critical times. Numerous lives have been touched, and Ann has deepened her roots in the Lord through her giving spirit.

Sandy was given a "courage stone" by a friend at the medical center. "It accompanied me to every surgery and to every chemo treatment," she recalls. "I had the opportunity to leave it with a friend I attended college with many years ago. He was facing prostate surgery—a much more frightening surgery, considering the potential loss, than mine was. It was emotional to leave that stone with Jack—he knew it, and so did I. What I did not leave there was my courage."

While the aftermath of cancer can go on for years, so too do the positive gains you made as a result of your journey through breast cancer. As Jane looks back on her cancer, she says, "Romans 8:28 actually is appropriate for me. I've seen a lot of 'good' come from my experiences. I developed a greater appreciation for simple things: the beauty of nature, the wind in my hair (now that I have hair again—you're sure you're the one whose hair won't grow back), the joy of family, less fear of dying, the ability to see things from more of an eternal perspective, a greater understanding of God's provision for me, and a witness to unbelievers that we don't have to face this alone."

The women I've treated who have a strong faith in God would add their hearty amens to Jane's list. Yes, breast cancer is hard. But, yes, breast cancer also comes bearing gifts from God.

What Loved Ones Can Do

Don't make an invalid out of your friend. Being as active as possible and doing as much as possible for herself can only do her good. We now know that bed is the worst place for a patient after surgery. Granted, energy levels are low, and naps may be needed. But recovery is much swifter and complications are reduced when the patient is up and active. This helps not only the body but also the mind. Just use common sense and help the patient to avoid getting overly tired.

When a patient comes home from the hospital, don't focus on her being ill. Focus instead on something fun with the family and let the treatment fall into the background. The few things that need to be attended to should take only a few minutes a day. Home health nurses are wonderful and needed in certain circumstances. But they play into the patient's own concept that "I'm sick." That mental attitude alone will prolong recovery. It's healthy for your friend to pamper herself a little during this time. But do something fun rather than focus on illness.

Be creative and specific in your offers of help for your friend. For example, if you are a masseuse, donate a session or two for your friend (and maybe her spouse). If you like to work out, consider doing it with your friend to support and encourage her efforts. Pick something you enjoy doing, and find a way to incorporate that into your friend's recovery.

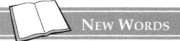 New Words

Lymphedema: A condition in which the lymphatic system has an accumulation of excess protein-containing lymphatic fluid in an affected extremity, causing fluid collection in tissue. This may occur after removal of lymph nodes.

Lymphocyte: A type of cell that constitutes 20 to 30 percent of the white blood cells of normal human blood. White blood cells' primary function is to combat infection.

Manual lymphatic drainage therapy: A massage treatment performed by applying a gentle massage in the direction of normal lymphatic flow. This massage stimulates the flow of lymphatic fluid through the lymphatic system and back to the bloodstream.

Phytochemicals: Food factors, found in fruits, vegetables, herbs, and other whole foods, that elicit profound effects on the maintenance of health and disease prevention.

Sequential pump: A machine that inflates and deflates air chambers in a device that is wrapped around the arm to help move the fluid that causes arm swelling from the arm toward the shoulder.

STRENGTHENING THOUGHTS FROM GOD'S WORD

"But those who hope in the Lord will renew their strength. They will soar on wings like eagles; they will run and not grow weary, they will walk and not be faint" (Isa. 40:31).

"Restore us to yourself, O Lord, that we may return; renew our days as of old" (Lam. 5:21).

"Put on the new self, which is being renewed in knowledge in the image of its Creator" (Col. 3:10).

CHAPTER 14

AFTER CANCER

My nurse, Deborah, actively supports our patients, coaching and cheerleading them through their breast cancer journeys. Part of the reason she's so good at what she does is that she, too, is a breast cancer survivor. I want to close with her thoughts on how breast cancer touched her life. Here's her story:

"What was I like before breast cancer? I was a workaholic. I worked every shift I could get. My plan was to retire by age 40 and live the easy life.

"Meanwhile, I was a super mom. I volunteered for everything. Bake 500 cookies, laminate fifty papers, work in the school nurse's office, take twelve Girl Scouts on a field trip, and help with homework all in the next ten hours? Sure!

"And I was an immaculate housekeeper. Everything was in its place all the time. Vacuum, dust, laundry, and scrub—that was my daily routine. Always planning, making lists, everything was on a schedule.

"Now, you might find this hard to believe, but what I'm about to say is the truth. Cancer was one of the best things that ever happened to me.

"Shortly after my diagnosis, I had worked my third night in a row, each shift being twelve to thirteen hours on a cardiac floor (a very demanding floor to work on) at Baylor University Medical Center. I had a PTA meeting—which I never missed—in forty-five minutes. As I drove home, which took thirty minutes on a busy highway, I calculated whether I would have enough time to shower to look perfect. I was running behind schedule.

"Then, over the highway I saw a beautiful object. Then another and another. I stopped the car and got out as other vehicles sped by. I climbed on the hood of my car and leaned back on the windshield. For more than an hour I watched a kaleidoscope of different-shaped hot air balloons float by. I missed the meeting. I did not vacuum that day. I declined when my job called me to work that night.

"You see, I wasn't alone on the hood of the car that day. Jesus was beside me. He had been waiting patiently for years for me to slow down and to visit with him. My cancer caused me to take a new view of life, and when I paused long enough to listen to God, he gave me a new peace, a new purpose. My conversations with my Father changed me after that day. I abandoned some major distractions in my life—my desire to make enough money to retire, my drive to be the best, my worry about what others thought, my stressing over all the tomorrows.

"Cancer taught me I didn't know if I had a tomorrow. Cancer taught me that true hope and love were based on confidence in God and on faith, not on egotistical plans for the future. Cancer taught me not to be overly optimistic about what I could do and what I could control. Instead it taught me to expect tribulation. Because cancer is tribulation—but it's a tribulation that taught me character.

Cancer taught me to walk with God by involving my mind, my heart, and my will in that relationship. I learned that even though previously I had the Lord as my Savior, I had missed the best part, the relationship.

"In the past God had always blessed me with peace when I needed to make a decision, but I had something more precious now. I had long-standing peace because I had surrendered everything to his loving control."

Deborah had learned that the one who cared the most about her during her journey through cancer wasn't her family or her friends or even herself; it was God. May that same truth be vividly apparent to you as you journey through breast cancer. May this "tribulation" bring you blessed relief from all the earthly distractions that have kept you from experiencing the wonder of being cared for by your Father God, the great Caregiver.

RISK FACTORS

The incidence of breast cancer has risen by about 1 percent annually in the United States over the past fifty years, with that rate of increase slowing over the past decade. We know that industrialized nations have a higher incidence than nonindustrialized regions of the world, but the reason is elusive. Higher fat intake or other environmental factors don't seem to hold the explanation. Chemicals such as pesticides have been studied, also without a clear association with breast cancer.

Although it's helpful to be informed about breast cancer risk factors, the significance is often misunderstood. Most women who develop breast cancer have no recognized risk factors, and most women who do have a risk factor, such as a family history, don't develop breast cancer.

Risk factors represent large population trends, but on an individual basis, they can't predict whether a particular woman will develop breast cancer.

Keeping all that in mind, let's talk about the risk factors.

Sex and Age

The most significant factor is being female, even though some men do develop breast cancer. We also know that the incidence of breast cancer increases with age. Approximately 75 percent of breast cancer occurs in women age 50 or older.

Family History

Our understanding of the role genes play in the risk of breast cancer is rapidly increasing. The genes reside in the cell nucleus and are part of the cell's DNA. Probably about 5 percent of breast cancer cases occur in women with a mutation of BRCA1, BRCA2, or other genes, which can be inherited from either the maternal or paternal side of the family. Testing for a mutation is becoming more available and may be useful in families with multiple cases of breast and ovarian cancer. But breast cancer can cluster in families without any genetic cause, perhaps related to environmental or lifestyle factors they have in common. In general, the younger the occurrence of breast cancer, the more likely a genetic factor may have been involved.

A first-degree relative (mother, sister, daughter) is a stronger risk factor than second-degree relatives (aunts, grandmothers, or cousins). The number of relatives involved and their ages also impact a woman's risk, as well as family history of ovarian cancers and other malignancies. The weight of these family risk factors in determining an individual woman's risk of breast cancer is the focus of ongoing research.

Hormonal Factors

No pregnancy, late first pregnancy (after age 30), early menarche (onset of menstrual periods), and late menopause all affect natural estrogen and progesterone levels. The years of exposure to these hormones is thought to influence the risk of breast cancer.

Oral Contraceptives

More than fifty studies have looked at the possible association of oral contraceptives with breast cancer, but most of them have shown little or no association. In those studies showing an increased risk of breast cancer, the risk seemed to be greater in women who were young (under 20) at the time they began using oral contraceptives, and who had prolonged use over ten years.[1] Information about women taking oral contraceptives who have other risk factors such as a family history is sparse and inconclusive, but no additional risk is suggested.

Contraceptives that use progesterone only, such as Norplant and Depo-Provera, have received limited research in relation to breast cancer risk. No increased risk has been demonstrated in the information currently available.[2]

Hormone Replacement Therapy

Hormone replacement therapy after menopause has been a topic of much research since the 1960s. Several solid studies in the past few years have offered increasing evidence of an association of combined estrogen and progesterone with a slightly increased risk of breast cancer.[3] But a combination of estrogen and progesterone is beneficial for preventing uterine cancer in women with a uterus. A study combining data from fifty-one studies showed a 14 percent increase in breast cancer among women who had ever used estrogen.[4] This increased risk was seen mostly in women who were not obese. Overall, evidence indicates that risk increases with years of use and with current users. But the risk appears to diminish after estrogen and progesterone are discontinued.

One large study of 16,000 women reported in 2002 found that the combination of estrogen and progesterone might slightly increase the risk of breast cancer.[5] That study didn't confirm an increased risk among women taking estrogen alone. Although this study reported that for 10,000 women taking the combination for a year, eight new cancers could be caused, this number isn't an exact figure. Because the number of women in this study that developed breast cancer is small, the actual number of cases of breast cancer caused by the combination of estrogen and progesterone could be from zero to sixteen. Information like this is useful in pointing out that more research is needed and caution is necessary, but it isn't so conclusive that a woman should stop taking hormone replacement.

BREAST-FEEDING

Breast-feeding has not consistently been associated with decreased risk. In a review of thirty-two studies, half showed some decreased risk of breast cancer, particularly with prolonged breast-feeding.

MISCARRIAGE OR ABORTION

Spontaneous and induced abortions have been the focus of research in relation to the risk of breast cancer. A combined review of twenty-eight published reports showed a slight increase in breast cancer risk among women after abortion. Why this would be the case is unknown, but one theory is that pregnancy causes rapid growth of the breast tissue cells that produce milk. Early in the pregnancy, these cells divide rapidly and do not become fully mature until late in the pregnancy. If this process is suddenly interrupted, these cells don't mature properly and may therefore be more susceptible to forming cancer.

Because abortion is a sensitive topic, one criticism of most of these studies is that the true incidence of abortion in the breast cancer group versus the group without breast cancer may be inaccurate. One very large study from Denmark found an increased incidence of breast cancer only in women having abortions in the second trimester.[6]

OTHER FACTORS

ALCOHOL

Alcohol consumption has a weak association with breast cancer incidence. In a combined review of thirty-eight studies, a consistent trend of a slightly increased risk of breast cancer in women drinking alcohol daily was shown. Recent alcohol consumption may have a stronger correlation to breast cancer risk than drinking patterns earlier in life. The more drinks per day, the higher the breast cancer risk, but overall, this is a weak risk factor.

HIGH FAT INTAKE

High fat intake in economically affluent countries has been a suspected culprit in the incidence of breast cancer. But after many animal and population studies, no clear association has been substantiated. Anything common in these industrialized countries could be the culprit, such as chemicals, inadequate exercise, and delayed childbearing.

OBESITY

Obesity may be a risk factor in postmenopausal women. In premenopausal women, some studies have suggested a decreased risk of breast cancer in obese women, with the risk increasing after menopause. But in non-Western countries, an increased incidence is shown in obese postmenopausal women, but no decrease in pre-menopausal women.[7] The relationship of body height and weight to breast cancer is complex and still being studied.

CAFFEINE

Caffeine consumption is not associated with increased risk of breast cancer, but it may have some effect on benign breast conditions such as breast tenderness.

RADIATION

Radiation exposure information has been gleaned from Hiroshima population studies as well as from women treated many years ago with high radiation exposure for other conditions such as tuberculosis. These studies show that adolescent women are most susceptible to damage from exposure to radiation and to increased risk of breast cancer years later. The dose of radiation used to obtain a mammogram is several orders of magnitude lower than that needed to cause cancer. A woman can obtain hundreds, if not thousands, of mammograms without significantly increasing her risk of breast cancer.

CHEMICALS

Chemicals such as pesticides have been the focus of numerous studies. The results have been mixed, but the combined information suggests no association or only a very weak association with breast cancer.[8]

ELECTROMAGNETIC FIELDS

Electromagnetic field exposure from power lines, electricity transformers, and even electric appliances has been studied. It is difficult to accurately study this possible risk because levels of exposure depend on indirect estimates and recall. Large population studies with mapping of residential wiring have not confirmed any association.[9] Use of electric blankets produced prior to 1990 has suggested a weak association with breast cancer in a couple of studies, but several others showed no association.[10] It's unlikely this plays a significant role.

SILICONE BREAST IMPLANTS AND UNDERWIRE BRAS

Silicone breast implants and underwire bras don't increase the risk of breast cancer. Nor do antiperspirants or aluminum compounds.

SMOKING

Smoking hasn't been associated with an increased risk of breast cancer.

GEOGRAPHIC LOCATION

Geographic location influences breast cancer risk. Population studies show that the United States and northern European countries have the highest incidence of breast cancer, with the lowest in Asian countries. Immigrants to the United States from low-risk countries may develop an increased incidence of breast cancer within one or two generations.[11]

STRESS

Stress affects the immune system, but by itself does not cause breast cancer. In one study, well-educated women often felt they were responsible for their development of breast cancer because of stress in their lives.[12]

REDUCING RISK

Some studies have been done to attempt to locate factors or lifestyle changes that could reduce the risk of breast cancer.

VITAMINS

Dietary factors such as high fiber and vitamins A, C, and E have all been studied in relation to their potential to reduce risk of breast cancer. With the exception of vitamin A, which may decrease breast cancer risk, none of these other factors has shown a consistent benefit in reducing breast cancer.

PHYSICAL EXERCISE

Physical exercise has also been studied. This is a particularly important issue, since it's a lifestyle choice that can be modified. More than seventeen published studies show an overall trend toward lower breast cancer risk in women who are physically active. This factor may be most important in younger women under 40 years of age.[13]

SOY

Phytoestrogens (estrogen-like compounds derived from plant sources) and soy products are the focus of both scientific and popular attention. Not enough research has been done to know what effect these have on breast cancer risk.[14]

A RISK FORMULA

A large study of women at above-average risk for breast cancer has used a formula developed by Mitchell H. Gail at the National Cancer Institute (NCI) to correctly predict the number of women who would develop breast cancer over several years.[15] Dr. Gail developed the formula in 1989 based on the incidence of breast cancer among women enrolled in a large screening study (called the BCDDP project) carried out in the 1970s. It has been used to accurately predict the number of breast cancers that would develop in several study groups. While we can't predict whether a particular woman will develop breast cancer, the formula is useful for obtaining an approximation of an individual woman's risk.

In most cases, women are surprised to find that their risk is lower than they had thought. A 30-year-old Caucasian woman who started her menstrual cycle at age 12, had her first pregnancy at age 20, and whose mother had breast cancer would have a calculated two in 1,000 chance of developing breast cancer in the next five years, and a lifetime risk of about 19 percent if she had no previous breast biopsies. That same woman would have a one in 1,000 risk over the next five years if her mother had not had breast cancer. The same woman at 45 years of age would have a sixteen in 1,000 chance of developing breast cancer in the next five years if her mother had breast cancer and five in 1,000 if her mother did not have breast cancer.

The Gail model uses only a few of the known risk factors, such as the age menstrual periods started, current age, close (mother or sister) family history of breast cancer, and previous breast biopsies. This model will be refined further and is a helpful first step in quantifying the risk of breast cancer.

As you can see, much more research needs to be done to pinpoint the causes of—and prevention of—breast cancer.

Appendix B

Resources

Organizations

American Cancer Society

www.cancer.org

By phone: (800) 227-2345

By mail: American Cancer Society National Home Office, 1599 Clifton Road, Atlanta, GA 30329

American Society of Clinical Oncology

www.asco.org

By phone: (703) 299-0150

By mail: 1900 Duke Street, Suite 200, Alexandria, VA 22314

Avon Breast Cancer Foundation

www.avoncrusade.com

By mail: Avon Breast Cancer Crusade, 1345 Avenue of the Americas, New York, NY 10105

Breastcancer.org

www.breastcancer.org (An online, nonprofit organization)

The Breast Cancer Resource Committee

www.afamerica.com/bcrc/index.htem

By phone: (202) 463-8040; Fax: (202) 463-8015

By mail: 2005 Belmont Street NW, Washington, DC 20009

Breast Cancer Society of Canada

www.bcsc.ca

By phone: (800) 567-8767

By mail: 401 St. Clair Street, Point Edward, ON, Canada N7V1P2

Canadian Breast Cancer Network

www.cbca.ca

By phone: (800) 685-8820

By mail: Suite 602, 331 Cooper Street, Ottawa, ON, Canada,
         K2P0G5

Centers for Disease Control and Prevention

www.cdc.gov

By phone: (404) 639-3534

Coalition of National Cancer Cooperative Groups

www.cancertrialshelp.org

By phone: (877) 520-4457

Department of Veteran Affairs

www.va.gov

By phone: (202) 273-5400 (Washington, DC office)

Toll free: (800) 827-1000 (reaches local Virginia office)

By mail: Veterans Health Association, 810 Vermont Avenue
         NW, Washington, DC 20420

Gilda's Club

www.gildasclub.org

By phone: (888) 445-3248

Health Insurance Association of America

www.hiaa.org

By phone: (202) 824-1600

By mail: 555 13th Street NW, Suite 600, East Washington, DC
20004-1109

Health Resources and Services Administration

Hill-Burton Program

www.hrsa.gov/0sp/dfcr/about/aboutdiv.htm

By phone: (301) 443-5656

Toll free: (800) 638-0742. If calling from the Maryland area:
(800) 492-0359

By mail: Health Resources and Services Administration, U.S.
Department of Health and Human Services, Park
Lawn Building, 5600 Fishers Lane, Rockville, MD
20857

National Alliance of Breast Cancer Organizations

www.nabco.org

By phone: (888) 80-NABCO; (888) 806-2226

By mail: 9 East 37th Street, New York, NY 10016

National Breast Cancer Coalition

www.natlbcc.org

By phone: (800) 622-2838

By mail: 1707 L Street NW, Suite 1060, Washington, DC 20036

National Cancer Institute

www.nci.nih.gov

By phone: (301) 435-3848 (Public Information Office line)

By mail: National Cancer Institute Public Information Office, Bldg. 31, Room 10A31, 31 Center Drive, MSC 2580, Bethesda, MD 20892-2580

National Lymphedema Network

www.lymphnet.org

By phone: (800) 541-3259

By mail: National Lymphedema Network, Latham Square, 1611 Telegraph Avenue, Suite 1111, Oakland, CA 94612-2138

Susan G. Komen Foundation, The

www.komen.org

By phone: (800) IMAWARE; (800) 462-9273

By mail: 5005 LBJ Freeway, Suite 250, Dallas, TX 75244

Susan Love MD.com

www.susanlovemd.com

By phone: (310) 230-1712

By mail: Box 846, Pacific Palisades, CA 90272

United Seniors Health Cooperative

www.unitedseniorshealth.org

By phone: (202) 479-6973

Toll free: (800) 637-2604

By mail: USHC, Suite 200, 409 Third Street SW, Washington, DC 20024

Y-ME National Breast Cancer Organization

www.y-me.org

By phone: (800) 221-2141

By mail: 212 W. Van Buren, Suite 500, Chicago, IL 60607

Specific Topics

Breast reconstruction

The American Society of Plastic and Reconstructive Surgeons and Plastic Surgery Educational Foundation offers a site (www.plasticsurgery.org/surgery/brstrec.htm) about the process of breast reconstruction; www.breastdiseases.com/pe11.htm explains the different types of breast reconstruction and procedures.

Chemotherapy

Information about chemotherapy and hormonal therapy, including information on financial assistance: www.cancersupportive care.com/pharmacy.html.

Children

Harpham, Wendy S. *When a Parent Has Cancer: A Guide to Caring for Your Children.* New York: HarperCollins, 1997.

Harpham, Wendy S., Laura Numeroff, and David M. McPhail. *The Hope Tree: Kids Talk About Breast Cancer.* New York: Simon and Schuster, 2001.

Clinical trials

National Cancer Institute's Cancer Trials site lists current clinical trials that have been reviewed by NCI: cancertrials.nci.nih.gov.

Diet and nutrition (Cancer Prevention)

USDA Dietary Guidelines: www.usda.gov/cnpp.

Faith resources

Simmons, C. B. *Little Mo's Legacy: A Mother's Lessons, A Daughter's Story.* Irving, Tex.: Tapestry Press, 2001.

Sorge, B. *Secrets of the Secret Place: Keys to Igniting Your Personal Time with God.* Oasis House, P.O. Box 127, Greenwood, MO. 64034.

FAMILY RESOURCES

www.kidscope.org is a website designed to help children understand and deal with the effects of cancer on a parent.

Men's Crusade Against Breast Cancer: home.earthlink.net/rkupbens/mcabc is a resource for husbands and other family members that provides support, ways to cope, and promotion of research.

FINANCIAL RESOURCES

Medicaid information: http://www.hcfa.gov/medical/medicaid.htm

Family and Medical Leave Act: www.dol.gov/dol/esa/public/regs/statues/whd/fmla.htm

Health Care Financing Administration's (HCFA) information website about breast cancer and medical programs: www.hcfa.gov/medicaide/bccpt/default/htm

www.needymeds.com offers information about programs sponsored by pharmaceutical manufacturers to help people who cannot afford to purchase necessary drugs.

The National Financial Resource Book for Patients: A State-by-State Directory: www.data.patientadvocate.org

HAIR LOSS

Look Good, Feel Better program through local American Cancer Society offices or (800) 395-LOOK.

"Buyer's Guide to Wigs and Hairpieces." This two-page summary, as well as additional literature, is available from Ruth L. Weintraub Co., 420 Madison Avenue, Suite 406, New York, NY 10017; phone (212) 838-1333.

HORMONAL THERAPY

National Cancer Institute's Fact Sheet "Questions and Answers about Tamoxifen," http://www.cis.nci.nih.gov/fact/7_16.htm; also, "Understanding Estrogen Receptors, Tamoxifen, and Raloxifene," www.rex.nci.nih.gov/behindthenews.uest.uestframe.htm

Frequently asked questions about Tamoxifen: www.cancersupportivecare.com/tamoxifen.html

LYMPHEDEMA

National Lymphedema Network: www.lymphnet.org

MAMMOGRAPHY INFORMATION

American College of Radiology/Radiological Society of North America gives a detailed discussion of what mammography is, step-by-step explanation of the procedure, and pictures of the equipment, answering questions about the safety and comfort of the procedure: www.radiologyinfo.org/content/mammogram.htm.

MALE BREAST CANCER

www.Interact.withus.com/interact/mbc/about/htm

The Susan G. Komen Foundation: Male Breast Cancer, www.breastcancerinfo.com/bhealth.html.male_breast_cancer.asp.

METASTATIC BREAST CANCER

Resource center solely for patients with metastatic breast cancer: www.patientcenters.com/breastcancer

MINORITIES AND BREAST CANCER

The Breast Cancer Resource Committee seeks to educate African-American women about breast cancer: www.afamerican.com/bcrc/index.htm

National Asian Women's Health Organization

www.nawho.org/womens_health/bcc_program.html

By phone: (415) 989-9747

By mail: 250 Montgomery Street, Suite 900, San Francisco, CA 94104

The Living Beyond Breast Cancer Foundation

www.ibbc.org/outreach.asp offers a complimentary book for African-American women, *Getting Connected: African-Americans Living Beyond Breast Cancer*

www.cancerlinks.org/breast.html#ETHNIC offers a listing of breast cancer websites for ethnic groups.

www.blackwomenshealth.com has a section dealing with breast cancer.

MISINFORMATION ABOUT BREAST CANCER

Specific debunking of the antiperspirant myth: www.pathguy. com/antipers.htm

NAUSEA/VOMITING

National Comprehensive Cancer Network: www.nccn.org/ patient_guidelines/Nausea-and-vomiting/nausea-and-vomiting/ 1_introduction.htm

Royal Marsden Hospital Patient Information On Line: www.royalmarsden.org/patientinfo/booklets/coping/nausea7.asp #heading

PREGNANCY

The National Cancer Institute has up-to-date information dealing with pregnancy and breast cancer, including treatment options, information about breast-feeding, etc.: www.cancer.gov

MD Anderson Cancer Center has a protocol regarding pregnancy and breast cancer: www.mdanderson.org/diseases/breast cancer.pregnancy

RADIATION THERAPY

National Cancer Institute/CancerNet: *Radiation Therapy and You: A Guide to Self-Help During Cancer Treatment,* www.cancer.gov
By phone: (800) 422-6237 (in English and Spanish)

RISK ASSESSMENT

National Cancer Institute's Risk Assessment Tool: www.cancer.gov/cancerinfo/doc.aspx?viewid=16c773e8-dd68-4ab8-a8eb-2fced63d41d6

SUPPORT GROUPS

National Alliance of Breast Cancer Organization listing of support groups by state: www.nabco.org/support

TERMINOLOGY

Glossary of Breast Cancer Terms: www.cancerhelp.com/ed/glossary.htm
Breast Cancer Glossary: www.breastcancer.about.com/library/glossary/blglossar.htm?terms=breast+cance

TREATMENT LOCATORS: PHYSICIANS AND HOSPITALS

AIM DocFinder (State Medical Board Executive Directors): a nonprofit organization providing a health professional licensing database. www.docboard.org

AMA Physician Select (American Medical Association): AMA database of demographic and professional information on individual physicians in the United States. www.ama-assn.org/aps/amahg.htm

American Board of Medical Specialties provides verification of physician qualifications and a list of specialists.

www.abms.org

By phone: (866) ASK-ABMS or American Board of Medical Specialties

By mail: 1007 Church Street, Suite 404, Evanston, IL 60201-5913

Hospital Select (American Medical Association & Medical-Net, Inc.): Hospital locator database searchable by hospital name, city, state, or zip code. Hospital Select data includes basic information: beds and utilization; service lines; and accreditation: www.hospitalselect.com/curb_db/owa/sp_hospselect.main

Directory of NCI-designated Cancer Centers. Fifty-eight research-oriented U.S. institutions recognized for scientific excellence and extensive cancer resources. www.cancertrials.nci.nih.gov/finding/centers/html/map.html

The National Comprehensive Cancer Network (NCCN) is an alliance of leading cancer centers. Members provide the highest quality in cancer care and cancer research. Each listing features phone numbers, website links, and a brief summary of website resources.

www.nccn.org

By phone: (888) 909-6226

NOTES

Chapter 1: The Journey Begins
1. Joseph Bayly, *The Last Thing We Talk About* (Elgin, Ill.: Cook, 1973).

Chapter 4: Consulting the Great Physician
1. Keith Willhite, "Lessons Along a Detour," *Moody Magazine* (September–October 2001): 44–47.
2. Ibid., 44.
3. Ibid., 46.
4. Ibid., 47.
5. Ibid.
6. Danny Houze, "Petition: Bring Our Community Together," *Kindred Spirit* (Summer 2002).

Chapter 6: Choosing the Right Surgery for You
1. D. A. Winchester, J. M. Jeske, and R. A. Goldschmidt, "The Diagnosis and Management of Ductal Carcinoma In-Situ of the Breast," *CA Cancer Journal Clinic* 50 (May–June 2000): 184–200.

Chapter 7: The Next Step
1. "Early Breast Cancer Trialists' Collaborative Group: Polychemotherapy for Early Breast Cancer: An Overview of the Randomized Trials," *Lancet* 352, no. 9132 (September 1998): 930–42.
2. G. Bonadonna and G. P. Valagussa, "Dose-Response Effect of Adjuvant Chemotherapy in Breast Cancer," *New England Journal of Medicine* 304, no. 1 (January 1981): 10.
3. B. Fisher, R. G. Ravdin, and R. K. Ausman, "Surgical Adjuvant Chemotherapy in Cancer of the Breast: Results of a Decade of Cooperative Investigation," *Annals of Surgery* 168 (1968): 337.

4. D. R. Budman and others, "Dose and Dose Intensity as Determinants of Outcome in the Adjuvant Treatment of Breast Cancer," *Journal of the National Cancer Institute* 90, no. 16 (August 1998): 1205–11.

5. S. Rodenhuis and others, "A Randomized Trial of High-Dose Chemotherapy and Hematopoietic Progenitor-Cell Support in Operable Breast Cancer with Extensive Axillary Lymph-Node Involvement," *Lancet* 352, no. 9127 (August 1998): 470; G. N. Hortobagyi, A. U. Buzdar, and R. Champlin, "Lack of Efficacy of Adjuvant High-Dose Tandem Combination Chemotherapy for High Risk Primary Breast Cancer—A Randomized Trial," *Proceedings of the American Society of Clinical Oncology* 17 (1998): 471.

6. Debasish Tripathy, "Oncogene-Directed Therapy: A Positive Message with a Cautionary Note," *Breast Diseases* (2000).

7. C. K. Osborne and P. M. Ravdin, "Adjuvant Systemic Therapy in Primary Breast Cancer," *Diseases of the Breast* 2d ed. (2000).

Chapter 8: Moving Onward: Radiation Therapy

1. B. C. Fisher and others, "Eight-Year Results of a Randomized Clinical Trial Comparing Total Mastectomy and Lumpectomy with or without Irradiation in the Treatment of Breast Cancer," *New England Journal of Medicine* 320, no. 13 (May 1989): 822–28.

2. F. Baclesse, "Roentgen Therapy Alone in Cancer of the Breast," *Acta Un Int Cancer* 15 (1959): 102–3.

3. E. D. Montague and others, "Conservative Surgery and Irradiation as an Alternative to Mastectomy in the Treatment of Clinically Favorable Breast Cancer," *CANCER*, 54, no. 11 (December 1984): 2668–72.

Chapter 9: Alternative Healing Methods

1. Walt Larimore and Donal O'Mathuna, *Alternative Medicine: The Christian Handbook* (Grand Rapids: Zondervan, 2001).

Chapter 12: Helping Children Face the Challenge

1. Cindy Brinker Simmons, *Little Mo's Legacy: A Mother's Lessons, A Daughter's Story* (Irving, Tex.: Tapestry, 2001), 63.

Appendix A: Risk Factors

1. "Collaborative Group on Hormonal Factors in Breast Cancer. Breast cancer and hormonal contraceptives: collaborative reanalysis of individual data on 53,297 women with breast cancer and 100,239 women without breast cancer—from 54 epidemiologic studies," *Lancet* 47 (1996): 1713–27.

2. WHO Collaborative Study of Neoplasia and Steroid Contraceptives, "Breast Cancer and Depot-Medroxyprogesterone Acetate: A Multinational Study," *Lancet* 338 (1991): 833–38.

3. K. K. Steinberg and others, "A Meta-Analysis of the Effect of Estrogen Replacement Therapy on the Risk of Breast Cancer," *Journal of the American Medical Association* 265 (1991): 1985–90; M. Sillero-Arenas and others, "Menopausal Hormone Replacement Therapy and Breast Cancer: A Meta-Analysis," *Obstetrics and Gynecology* 79 (1992): 286–94; J. Russo and I. H. Russo, "The Etiopathogenesis of Breast Cancer Prevention," *Cancer Lett* 90 (1995): 81–89.

4. "Collaborative Group on Hormonal Factors in Breast Cancer. Breast cancer and hormone replacement therapy: collaborative reanalysis of data from 51 epidemiologic studies of 52,705 women with breast cancer and 108,411 women without breast cancer," *Lancet* 350 (1997): 1047–59.

5. Initiative Women's Health, "Risks and Benefits of Estrogen Plus Progestin in Healthy Postmenopausal Women," *Journal of the American Medical Association* 288 (2002): 321–33.

6. J. Brind and others, "Induced Abortions as an Independent Risk Factor for Breast Cancer: A Comprehensive Review and Meta-Analysis," *Journal of Epidemiology and Community Health* 50 (1996): 481–96; M. Melbye, J. Wohlfahrt, and J. Olsen, "Induced Abortion and the Risk of Breast Cancer," *New England Journal of Medicine* 336 (1997): 81–85.

7. M. P. Longnecker, "Alcoholic Beverage Consumption in Relation to Risk of PBC: Meta-Analysis and Review," *Cancer Causes Control* 5 (1994): 73–82.

8. W. C. Willett, B. Rockhill, and S. E. Hankinson, "Epidemiology and Nongenetic Causes of Breast Cancer," in J. R. Harris and others, eds., *Diseases of the Breast,* 2d ed. (Philadelphia: Lippincott & Williams, 2000).

9. Ibid.

10. M. D. Gammon and others, "Electric Blanket Use and Breast Cancer Risk Among Younger Women," *American Journal of Epidemiology* 148 (1998): 556–63.

11. J. Russo and I. H. Russo, "The Etiopathogenesis of Breast Cancer Prevention," *Cancer Lett* 90 (1995): 81–89.

12. Ibid.

13. L. Bernstein and others, "Physical Exercise and Reduced Risk of Breast Cancer in Young Women," *Journal of the National Cancer Institute* 86, no. 18 (September 1994): 1403–08.

14. W. C. Willett, B. Rockhill, and S. E. Hankinson, "Epidemiology and Nongenetic Causes of Breast Cancer," J. R. Harris and others, eds., *Diseases of the Breast*, 2d ed. (Philadelphia: Lippincott & Williams, 2000).

15. M. H. Mitchell and others, "Projecting individualized probabilities of developing breast cancer for white females who are being examined annually," *Journal of the National Cancer Institute* 81 (January 1989): 1879–86.

ABOUT THE AUTHORS

Dr. Sally M. Knox is a breast cancer surgeon at Baylor Medical Center in Dallas, Texas. Trained in general surgery at St. Luke's Hospital in Kansas City, she took additional training specific to breast cancer treatment and has devoted her practice to helping women and families with breast cancer over the past 15 years. Early in her practice she became involved in helping women find resources and support in their journey through breast cancer and helped to found a non-profit organization specifically to assist under-insured women who find themselves battling this disease. Dr. Knox has also been involved in medical missions and training worship leaders in the former Soviet Union. She enjoys music, and experiencing the beauty of God's kingdom through hiking and biking. Her brother and sisters, as well as a niece, Ryan, provide a constant source of joy for her.

Janet Kobobel Grant collaborated on *Every Child Needs a Praying Mom* and several Women of Faith titles. She also has written Women of Faith Bible studies, *But Can She Type?* and *Where Is God When I Need Him Most?* A former managing editor for books at Focus on the Family, she makes her home in Santa Rosa, California, with her husband and their Australian shepherd, Murphy.

SCRIPTURE INDEX

Genesis
37   70

Exodus
2   70
14:21   66

Deuteronomy
31:6   149

2 Samuel
22:33   52

Job
12   70
42:5   65

Psalms
4:8   173
16:11   109, 149
27:13–14   140
31:24   149
33:20–22   140
33:22   109
34   158
34:1   173
46:10   35, 164
62:1   140
68:6   192
103:13   192
121   21
128:6   192
139:17   60
139:23   35
139:56   70

143:8   109
145:14   53
145:17–18   60

Proverbs
3:6   87
10:12   183
15:17   183
20:24   61
24:6   67, 69

Song of Solomon
2:34   183

Isaiah
26:3   164
40:31   207

Lamentations
5:21   207

Matthew
4   70
6:8   128
11:3   70
11:6   70
11:11   70
14   66, 67
19:26   173

John
3:16   62
9   66
14:12   67

Acts
7   70
14:19   70
16:25   57

Romans
3:23   62
5:8   62
8:28   53, 205

Ephesians
3:12   26
3:17–19   35

Colossians
3:10   207

2 Thessalonians
3:5   87

2 Timothy
1:7   53

Hebrews
4:16   128
10:35–36   26
12:2   57

Subject Index

A

abortion, 216–17
absolute differences, 123, 127
acceptance, 61–62, 100, 186
adjuvant therapy, 111, 127
Adriamycin, 144
alcohol, 217
alternative healing, 141–49
Alternative Medicine: The Christian Handbook, 143
aluminum compounds, 219
American Cancer Society, 29, 168
American College of Radiology, 29
anemia, 117
anger, 19, 153, 155–56, 160, 162, 169, 180, 188
antibiotics, 201–2
antidepressants, 159
antiestrogens, 125
antioxidants, 143, 144
antiperspirants, 219
aromatase inhibitors, 125
arthritis, 97
artificial breast, 82, 85
astralagus, 148
attitude, 48, 60–61, 68, 142, 156, 176, 191, 206
atypical duct hyperplasia, 134–35
axillary dissection, 77, 80, 81, 199

B

Bible, 62, 66–67, 100
biological-based therapies, 143–46
biopsies, 14, 31–34, 79–81, 199
birth control pills, 125, 215

black cohosh, 147
blinded study, 122–23, 127
blood cell count, 117
blood clots, 125
blood tests, 90, 103
bone density test, 197
bone marrow, 117
bone marrow research, 120–21
bone scan, 103, 104, 106
boost, 136–37, 140
breast cancer types, 92–95. *See also* cancer
breast-conserving therapy, 77–78
breast-feeding, 216
breast illustrations, 76, 80
breast implants, 96, 219
breast lobules, 78, 94
breast reduction, 96
breast size, 95–96
Brinker, Maureen Connolly, 190
burdock root, 146

C

caffeine, 218
calcium D-glucarate, 144
Camellia sinensis, 146
cancer
    "cause" of, 18–19
    detecting, 28–33
    discovery of, 13–18
    discussing, 23–24, 176, 178–80, 186–87
    early detection, 93–94
    following, 209–11
    increase in, 213

recovery from, 193–206
recurrence of, 94, 106, 135, 136
responses to, 14–17
types of, 92–95
understanding, 27–28
"why" of, 17–18, 53, 58–59, 163
cancer cells. *See* tumor cells
cancer centers, 41–42, 168
capsular contracture, 96, 106
carcinoma, 93–95, 105, 107, 134–35
career considerations, 118, 168–69
catheters, 117–18, 137, 140
celebrations, 138–40, 193, 194
checkups, 196–97
chemicals, 213, 218
chemotherapy
    course or cycle of, 113, 127
    definition of, 51
    explanation of, 113–14
    length of, 113
    need for, 78, 103–4
    physicians, 46
    preparation for, 118–20
    questions on, 118–19
    and reconstruction, 83
    research on, 114, 120–21
    response to, 118–19
    side effects of, 112
    suggestions for, 119–20
    support tips, 126–27
    treatments, 78, 96, 111–27
    chest wall radiation, 137–38
children
    communicating with, 23–24,
      186–87
    emotional problems, 186, 188
    feelings of, 23–24, 185–86
    help for, 185–92
    helping with, 191–92
    observing parents, 188–91
choices. *See* surgical options
church friends, 50–51, 166–68
clinical trials, 117, 122–24
coenzyme Q10, 143–44

collagen vascular disease, 97, 106
comfort, 21, 25–26, 56, 63–65, 162–
    63, 166–67
communication, 23–24, 176, 178–80,
    186–87
contraceptives, 125, 215
coping skills, 19–22, 155–56
core needle biopsy, 32–33, 34
Coumadin, 147
counselors
    interviewing, 49
    role of, 48–49
    support from, 161–62, 168
courage, 16, 154, 157, 191, 205
CT scans, 31, 103, 104
cyst aspiration, 31–33, 41
cysts, 31–32

D
David, 57, 70
death
    decrease in, 29, 160
    discussing, 157, 165, 170
decreased libido, 124, 198
deep vein clots, 125
denial, 156, 161–62, 166, 180–82
depression, 133, 147, 158–61, 165,
    169, 186
diagnostic mammogram, 30, 34. *See
    also* mammograms
diet, 119, 145–46, 197–98
Digoxin, 147
discussions, 23–24, 157, 165, 170,
    176, 178–80, 186–87
diuretics, 204
DNA, 18, 28, 130, 214
doctor appointments, 40–44
doctors. *See* medical team; physi-
    cians; surgeons
drug development, 122–25
duct cancer, 78, 86, 92–93
duct carcinoma in situ (DCIS), 93–
    94, 105
duct hyperplasia, 134–35

E

early detection, 93–94
Echinacea, 147
electromagnetic fields, 218–19
Elisha, 69
elm bark, 146
emotional fitness, 195–96
emotional healing, 24, 57–58, 155–62
emotions
    facing, 16–18, 153–73
    of family, 23–24, 164–66, 180–82,
        185–92
    see also specific emotions
essiac, 146
estrogen production, 117, 215
estrogen products, 198
estrogen receptor status, 105, 106,
    121, 124
examinations, 18, 31
exercises
    following surgery, 102–3
    to increase energy, 118
    and risk reduction, 220
exhaustion, 159, 165, 194. *See also*
    fatigue

F

fact-finding, 42–43. *See also* research
faith
    and medical treatment, 65–70
    relying on, 17, 19, 21, 210–11
    see also God; Jesus
family feelings, 23–24, 164–66, 180–
    82, 185–92
family history, 97, 214
family support. *See* support
fat intake, 217
fatigue, 103, 117, 118, 133, 194, 195,
    198. *See also* exhaustion
fear, 15, 19, 23–24, 153, 156–58, 160,
    165, 169, 188, 193–96
fibrosis, 97, 134, 140
fine needle aspiration (FNA), 31–33,
    34

fluid pills, 204
free radicals, 143
friends' support. *See* support

G

Gail, Mitchell H., 220–21
garlic, 146
genetic factors, 97–98, 214
genetic testing, 97, 214
geographic locations, 219
ginger, 146–47
Ginkgo biloba, 146
ginseng, 146
glucarate, 144
God
    belief in, 62
    focus on, 57–58
    and medical treatment, 65–70
    praying to, 62, 64
    purpose of, 62, 65, 69–71
    relying on, 17, 19, 21, 210–11
    strength from, 26, 35, 52–53, 55–
        72, 87, 109, 128, 140, 149, 154,
        164, 169, 173, 183, 192, 207,
        210–11
    trusting, 56–60, 70–71
green tea, 146
grief, 24, 155, 161–62, 169, 180
growth factor receptor, 121
guilt, 17, 43, 59, 163, 169, 181, 186,
    188, 194
gynecologist, 124

H

hair loss, 112, 115–16, 126–27, 129,
    189–90, 195
headaches, 117, 119
healing
    alternative healing, 141–49
    components of, 57–58
    emotional healing, 24, 57–58,
        155–62
    spiritual healing, 55–56, 65–70
    helping others, 191–92, 204–5,
        209–11

herbs
and medical care, 143, 148–49
types of, 146–49
warnings on, 146–47
Herceptin, 121
high fat intake, 217
historic controls, 121, 127
home health nurses, 39, 206
hormonal factors, 214–15
hormonal therapy
definition of, 51
need for, 104
physicians, 46
hormone blocker therapy
explanation of, 105
treatments, 111–27
hormone receptors, 105
hormone replacement therapy, 125, 215–16
hot flashes, 117, 124, 199
Houze, Pastor Danny, 63
husband
communicating with, 176, 178–80
and household roles, 177–78
needs of, 164–66, 180–82
relationship changes, 176–77
and sexual relationship, 178–80, 198–99
support for, 181–82
support from, 175–76

I
in situ cancer, 86, 93–94, 107
in situ stage, 93
infection
and lymphedema, 199–201, 206–7
vulnerability to, 77, 80, 117, 120
infiltrating duct cancer, 86, 92–93, 95, 107
infiltrating lobular carcinoma, 94, 107
information gathering, 20, 22, 40–45, 157. See also research

insomnia, 119, 172
insurance considerations, 41
intestinal changes, 115, 117
intraductal breast cancer, 93–94
intraductal carcinoma, 105
invasive cancer, 78–79, 86, 92–94
invasive duct cancer, 86, 92–94, 107
invasive lobular cancer, 94
invasive lobular carcinoma, 94
invasive tumor, 105

J
Jesus
and healing, 55–56, 65–67
relationship with, 55–58, 65–67, 70, 100, 159, 163–64, 210–11
Job, 70, 163
John the Baptist, 70
Joseph, 65, 70
journaling, 50

L
Larimore, Dr. Walt, 143
libido, 124, 178–80, 198–99
liver sonogram, 103, 104, 107
lobular carcinoma in situ (LCIS), 95, 107, 134–35
lobular neoplasia, 95
loss, 24, 70
lumpectomy
exercises following, 102–3
explanation of, 77, 81
factors regarding, 85–86, 90, 92, 94–99
and radiation, 135–37
lumps, 77, 92, 93, 94
lupus, 97
lymph nodes
biopsies, 79, 81
definition of, 86
explanation of, 77
illustration of, 80
involvement of, 105
number of, 80
removal of, 77, 79, 80, 81, 199

THE BREAST CANCER CARE BOOK

lymphatic channels, 199–200
lymphatic fluid, 199–200
lymphedema, 199–201, 206–7
lymphocyte, 199, 207

M
macrobiotic diets, 145–46
malignancy, 28, 95, 115, 130, 134
mammograms
  and diagnosis, 18, 92–93
  explanation of, 29–31
  following treatment, 197
  locations for, 30
  process of, 29
  reading, 30–31
  records of, 30–31
manual lymphatic drainage (MLD),
  203, 204, 207
margins, 77, 91, 92, 94
markers, 106, 107
massage, 179, 203, 207
mastectomy
  exercises following, 102–3
  factors regarding, 90, 94–99
  and radiation, 137–39
  surgical options, 76–83, 86
medical appointments, 40–44
medical centers, 41–42
medical conditions, 97
medical history, 97, 214
medical knowledge, 67–68
medical oncologists
  consulting, 119
  questions for, 114–15
  role of, 46–47, 112, 113
medical opinions, 22, 44
medical records, 30–31, 38–40, 131
medical team
  interviewing, 42–43
  roles of, 44–49
  selecting, 40–43, 51–52
  size of, 38
medullary carcinoma, 95
melatonin, 144

memory loss, 117
menopausal symptoms, 117, 124,
  198–99
menopause, 124, 215, 217–18
metastatic disease, 104, 105, 107
milk thistle, 147
minerals, 143–45. See also vitamins
miracles, 66–67
miscarriage, 216–17
modified radical mastectomy, 78–
  79, 81
Moses, 66, 70
moving forward, 18–19, 22
MRIs, 31
multicentric disease, 92
multifocal disease, 92, 107

N
Naaman, 68–69
National Cancer Institute (NCI),
  220–21
nausea, 112, 115, 119, 145, 147, 148
needle biopsy, 31–32, 34
negative thinking, 158
nipple reconstruction, 83, 96
node biopsy, 79–80, 81
noninvasive cancer, 78
numbness, 102
nurses, 38, 39, 40, 48, 54, 65, 206. See
  also medical team
nutrition, 119, 145–46, 197–98

O
obedience, 66–67
obesity, 217–18
O'Mathuna, Donal, 143
oncologists, 45–47, 112
open surgical biopsy, 32–33, 34
opinions, 22, 44, 98
oral contraceptives, 125, 215
organizations, 223–26
osteoporosis, 197

P
pathologists, 77, 91–92

pathology report, 101
Paul, 56, 57, 63, 70
pectoralis muscle, 78
pelvic exams, 197
pesticides, 213, 218
Pettigrew, Jan, 161
phase-three trials, 122–24
physical activity, 103. *See also* exercises
physical examinations, 18, 31
physical exercise, 220. *See also* exercises
physical fitness, 195
physicians
    interviewing, 42–43
    primary care physician, 44–45
    selecting, 40–43, 51–52
    see also medical team; surgeons
phytochemicals, 197, 207
phytoestrogens, 147, 199, 220
plants, 142, 146–49. *See also* herbs
plastic surgery, 47, 82. *See also* reconstructive surgery
port insertion, 117–18
positive thinking, 158
prayer group, 50–51, 166–68
pregnancy, 31, 97, 214, 216
pride, 69, 186
primary care physician, 44–45. *See also* physicians
professional support. *See* counselors
professional team. *See* medical team
progesterone production, 117, 215
progesterone receptor status, 105, 106, 124
prognosis, 62, 87, 93, 94, 104–5, 112
prophylactic mastectomy, 97–98, 107
prosthesis, 82, 85, 86
protocol, 113, 127
pumps, 204

R
radiation exposure, 138–39, 218

radiation oncologist
    consultation with, 96
    questions for, 131
    role of, 47, 130–31
radiation therapy
    definition of, 51
    dosages, 130, 135, 136
    end of, 138–39
    explanation of, 129–30
    and implants, 137, 140
    and lumpectomies, 90
    need for, 77–78, 130
    physicians, 47
    preparing for, 130–31
    and reconstruction, 83
    sensation of, 132–33
    side effects, 132–34, 138
    site of, 131–32, 137
    skin marks, 131–32
    and smoking, 138
    support during, 139–40
    treatments, 78–79, 96–97, 129–40
radical mastectomy, 78, 81
radioactive implants, 137, 140
randomized trials, 122, 127
Reach for Recovery, 168
reconstructive surgeons, 47
reconstructive surgery, 82–86, 96, 98, 99
records. *See* medical records
recovery, 193–206
    and checkups, 196–97
    emotional fitness, 195–96
    feelings about, 193–94
    and nutrition, 197–98
    physical fitness, 195
    questions about, 193–94
    road to, 76
    spiritual fitness, 194
    and stress reduction, 142
recurrences, 94, 106, 135, 136
red blood cells, 117
relative differences, 123, 127
research

conducting, 20, 22, 40–45, 157
participating in, 41, 114, 117, 122–24
resources, 223–32
rheumatoid arthritis, 97
rhubarb, 146
risk factors, 97–98, 213–21
risk formula, 220–21
risk reduction, 219–20

S

St. John's Wort, 147
scans, 31, 32, 103, 104, 106, 131
scleroderma, 97
screening mammogram, 30, 34. *See also* mammograms
second opinions, 22, 44, 98
selective estrogen receptor modulators (SERMs), 125
selenium, 144–45
self-pity, 60–61, 191
sentinel node biopsy, 79–81, 199
sequential pump, 204, 207
sexuality, 124, 178–80, 198–99
shark cartilage, 145
side effects
    discussing, 112, 119
    reducing, 113, 145, 147, 148
    types of, 115–17
Silas, 57
silicone breast implants, 96, 219
Simmons, Cindy Brinker, 190
Simonds, Randy, 63–64
Simonds, Valerie, 63–65
simple mastectomy, 78, 81
skeletal survey, 104
smoking, 219
sonograms, 31, 32, 103, 107
soul, 62, 70, 72
soy, 146, 199, 220
spiritual fitness, 194
spiritual growth, 38, 53, 61, 154–55
spiritual healing, 55–56, 65–70
spiritual journey, 55–72

spouse, 164–66. *See also* husband
stages, 104–5
staging, 87, 104–5
staging tests, 103–4
stem cell research, 120–21
Stephen, 70
stereotactic core needle biopsy, 32–33, 34
strength from God, 26, 35, 52–53, 55–72, 87, 109, 128, 140, 149, 154, 164, 169, 173, 183, 192, 207, 210–11
stress
    effects of, 133, 172, 198, 219
    handling, 43, 48–49, 99–100, 163, 176, 219
    reducing, 40, 142, 143
    suffering, 26, 56, 58–62, 164
    supplements, 148, 220. *See also* vitamins
support
    finding, 162–64
    for family, 23–24, 48–49, 71–72, 107–8, 164–66, 181–82
    from family, 34–35, 50–51, 53–54, 100, 107–9, 139–40, 169–72, 175–76
    from friends, 24–26, 34–35, 50–51, 53–54, 107–9, 139–40, 162–63, 169–72, 191–92, 206
    group support, 50–51, 161, 166–68
    personal support, 23–26, 34–35
    tips for, 23–26, 34–35, 53–54, 71–72, 100, 107–9, 126–27, 139–40, 162–64, 169–72, 206
surgeons
    interviewing, 42–43
    role of, 45–46
    selecting, 40–43, 51–52
    see also medical team; physicians
surgery
    day of, 101–2
    exercises following, 102–3
    and family members, 100–101
    preparing for, 99–101

questions on, 98–99, 100–101
recovery from, 102–3
staging, 104–5
staging tests, 103–4
see also surgical options
surgical biopsy, 32–33, 34
surgical oncologists, 45
surgical options
decision-making, 98–99
factors regarding, 89–98
questions on, 98–101
staging, 103–5
types of, 75–87
see also surgery
surgical questions, 98–101
swelling
in arm, 77, 80, 199–200
of breast, 96, 132, 134
remedies for, 200–204
systemic therapy, 111–12, 127

T
Tamoxifen, 124–25, 197
teas, 146–47
teenagers, 187
total mastectomy, 78, 81
treatment plan, 113
treatment regimen, 113
trust, 16, 19, 40, 43, 51, 53, 56–62, 68, 70–71, 100, 164, 177
tubular carcinoma, 95
tumor
aggressiveness of, 105–6
growth rate of, 106
size of, 103, 105

see also tumor cells
tumor cells
and chemotherapy, 103–4, 114, 121
explanation of, 27–28
growth of, 92, 94
and hormonal therapy, 103–4, 124
location of, 77, 79, 80, 93, 104, 138
migration of, 122, 136
presence of, 32, 104
and radiation therapy, 51, 77–78, 97, 129–30, 135–36
response of, 122

U
ultrasonography, 31, 34, 107

V
vaginal bleeding, 124
vaginal dryness, 124, 198
vegetarian diets, 145–46
vein clots, 125
vitamins, 142, 143, 146, 148, 220

W
weakness, 56–57, 61, 64–65, 145, 154, 167
weight reduction, 202
white blood cells, 117
"why" of cancer, 17–18, 53, 58–59, 163
wigs, 115–16, 161, 189
Willhite, Dr. Keith, 58–59, 60, 61
work schedules, 118, 168–69

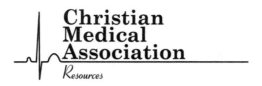

Christian Medical Association
Resources

Medically reliable ... biblically sound. That's the rock-solid promise of this dynamic new series offered by Zondervan and the Christian Medical Association. Because when your health is at stake, you can't settle for anything less than the whole truth.

Finally, people of faith can draw from both the knowledge of science and the wisdom of God's Word in addressing health care and medical ethics issues. This series allows you to benefit from cutting-edge knowledge of experienced, trusted, and respected medical scientists and practitioners. Now you can gain their insights into the vital interconnection of health and spirituality—a critical unity largely overlooked by secular science.

While integrating your faith and health can actually improve your physical well-being and even extend your life, it can also help you make health care decisions consistent with your beliefs. A sound biblical analysis of emerging treatments and technologies is essential to protecting yourself from seemingly harmless—yet spiritually, ethically, or medically unsound—options.

Founded in 1931, the Christian Medical Association helps thousands of doctors minister to their patients by imitating the Great Physician, Jesus Christ. Christian Medical Association members provide a Christian voice on medical ethics to policy makers and the media, minister to needy patients on medical missions around the world, evangelize and disciple students on more than 90 percent of the nation's medical school campuses, and provide educational and inspirational resources to the church.

To find out more about the Christian Medical Association's ministries and resources on health care and ethical issues, be sure to browse the website at www.christianmedicalassociation.org or call Christian Medical Association Life & Health Resources toll free at 888-231-2637.

> "Dear friend, I pray that you may enjoy good health and that all may go well with you, even as your soul is getting along well"(3 John 2 NIV).

When the Diagnosis Is Serious, What Makes the Difference Between Hope and Despair?

When Your Doctor Has Bad News

Simple Steps to Strength, Healing, and Hope

Al B. Weir, M.D., 2002–2003 President of the Christian Medical Association

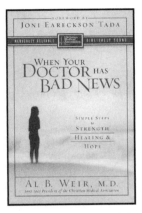

When Your Doctor Has Bad News offers no easy answers, no quick outs. But it does equip you to weather the storm you are facing and emerge whole again. Practical tips provide questions for you to ask your doctor and choices you can make to achieve your best chances for healing. Real-life stories show how others have coped with life-threatening illness, walked with God, and won.

A medical doctor with a pastor's heart, Dr. Weir knows from experience that it's the patient's focus, not the diagnosis that indicates whether one will slip into despair and hopelessness or have the courage to live each day fully. Resilience of spirit can powerfully influence recovery and healing, and within our crisis, the choices we make are important.

You can deepen communion with God in the midst of medical crisis. *When Your Doctor Has Bad News* gives you proven principles that will enable you to choose a life worth living, no matter what news the doctor has given you.

Softcover: 0-310-24742-X

Pick up a copy today at your favorite bookstore!

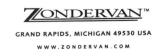

ZONDERVAN™

GRAND RAPIDS, MICHIGAN 49530 USA

WWW.ZONDERVAN.COM

10 Essentials of Highly Healthy People

*Walt Larimore, M.D.,
Host of Radio and TV's*
Focus on Your Family's Health,
with Traci Mullins

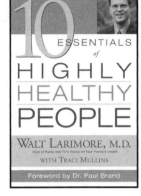

10 Essentials of Highly Healthy People is like having your very own health mentor to guide you in your total health picture, from treating illness and navigating the health-care system to developing a proactive approach to vibrant health.

You'll see how to balance the physical, emotional, relational, and spiritual parts of your life to help you achieve maximum health. Whether you're eighteen or eighty, you can become healthy—highly healthy.

- Master 10 powerful principles for improving your well-being.
- Discover the secret to becoming your own health-care quarterback.
- Chart your plan to improved health using the numerous self-assessments provided.
- Learn the right questions to ask your doctors.
- Gain the confidence to hire and fire your health-care providers.
- Explore the most reliable Internet resources available.

The 10 principles in this book have made a life-changing—and in many cases a life-saving—difference for countless people. They can for you too.

Hardcover: 0-310-24027-1

Pick up a copy today at your favorite bookstore!

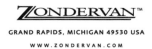

ZONDERVAN™

GRAND RAPIDS, MICHIGAN 49530 USA

WWW.ZONDERVAN.COM

New Light on Depression

Help, Hope, and Answers for the Depressed and Those Who Love Them

David B. Biebel, D.Min., and Harold G. Koenig, M.D.

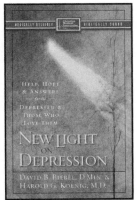

What is depression, really? A psychological disorder? An emotional problem? A case of negative self-talk? A spiritual weakness? Unresolved anger? A medical condition? How can it be successfully treated?

Whether you need a lifeline to cling to, knowledge to clear confusion, help determining the next step, or strength to help a loved one, *New Light on Depression* offers hope and healing. With understanding born of personal and professional experience, the authors—one a psychiatrist and the other a minister—untangle the web of depression.

Written for those who suffer from depression and those who want to help—family members, pastors, friends—this book equips you with the knowledge and tools to move toward a life of joy once more. It covers the full range of concerns, including the use of antidepressants. With personal applications, questions for reflection, and evaluation guides, *New Light on Depression* is a medically reliable and biblically sound resource for finding faith and strength in the midst of depression and emerging again whole and healthy.

Softcover: 0-310-24729-2

Pick up a copy today at your favorite bookstore!

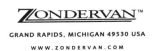

ZONDERVAN™

GRAND RAPIDS, MICHIGAN 49530 USA

WWW.ZONDERVAN.COM

Alternative Medicine

The Christian Handbook

*Dónal O'Mathúna, Ph.D.,
and Walt Larimore, M.D.*

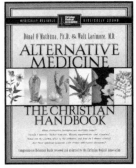

In today's health-conscious culture, options for the care and healing of the body are prolifer-ating like never before. But which ones can you trust? Some are effective, some are useless, some are harmful. Some involve forms of spirituality that the Bible expressly forbids. Others that are truly helpful have been avoided by some Christians who draw inaccurate conclusions about them.

Alternative Medicine is the first comprehensive guidebook to non-traditional medicine written from a distinctively Christian perspective. Here at last is the detailed and balanced coverage of alternative medicine that you've been looking for. Professor and researcher Dónal O'Mathúna, Ph.D., and national medical authority Walt Larimore, M.D., draw on their extensive knowledge of the Bible and their medical and pharmaceutical expertise to answer the questions about alternative medicine that you most want answered—and others you wouldn't have thought to ask.

Softcover: 0-310-23584-7

Pick up a copy today at your favorite bookstore!

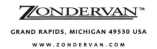

ZONDERVAN™

GRAND RAPIDS, MICHIGAN 49530 USA

WWW.ZONDERVAN.COM

We want to hear from you. Please send your comments about this book to us in care of zreview@zondervan.com. Thank you.

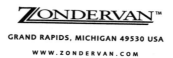

GRAND RAPIDS, MICHIGAN 49530 USA

WWW.ZONDERVAN.COM